GA
The He

Here are the facts about the remarkable medicinal properties of garlic, presenting the findings of recent research which support its age-old use as an antibiotic, antiseptic, blood cleanser and general tonic and describing its action against rheumatism, intestinal disorders, heart disease and even garden pests.

GARLIC
The Healing Herb

All about its remarkable range
of medicinal and culinary
properties

by

Paul Simons

THORSONS PUBLISHING GROUP

This edition first published 1986

British Library Cataloguing in Publication Data

Simons, Paul
Garlic.
1. Garlic — Therapeutic use — History
I. Title
615'.324'324   RM666.G15

ISBN 0 7225 1427 1

Published by Thorsons Publishers Limited, Denington Estate,
Wellingborough, Northants, NN8 2RQ

Printed in Great Britain by Richard Clay Limited,
Bungay, Suffolk

5   7   9   10   8   6

CONTENTS

INTRODUCTION

'Garlic then have power to save from death.
Bear with it though it maketh unsavoury breath,
and scorn not garlic like some that think, it
only maketh men wink and drink and stink.'

This quotation taken from *About Garlic* by G.J.
Binding (Thorsons) and attributed to an early
nineteenth-century writer, Sir John Harrington,
tells us a great deal about garlic. Its effect on the
breath of those who eat it is infamous. The
majority of people in the United Kingdom
consider its smell unsavoury, some would even
say anti-social, and yet in some parts of the
world the flavour of this humble herb is
generally revered for the subtle flavour it
imparts to a host of dishes, from simple stews
and soups to great culinary masterpieces.
However, the message that Sir John Harrington
so persuasively attempts to convey to his
readers is clear – certainly garlic makes the
breath smell, but this is well worth suffering in
order to obtain the benefits of its powerful
action as a natural remedy, effective against a
wide variety of diseases.

In Sir John's day there was no alternative to
the 'unsavoury breath'. Today, however, you
can purchase capsules containing the pure oil
of garlic, which dissolve in the small intestine,
thus eliminating the worst of the anti-social
disadvantages of garlic. They can be purchased
from any health food store.

No one knows when or how herbs first came
to be used to treat disease. Almost certainly it
was the primitive savages roaming the primeval

rain forests countless thousands of years ago who first came to understand that, when they ate certain plants or parts of a plant, their ailments were cured. It was accident, not research, that prompted the experiments which led to their use and it was instinct for survival not scientific knowledge that led them to pass on by word of mouth the benefits they had discovered, for the use of future generations. We do not really know how long ago, where or how the benefits of garlic were first discovered but our knowledge of its medicinal use does begin with the very first records kept by man.

Some of the very first writings of the early civilizations of Egypt, China, Greece and Rome, contain numerous references to the medicinal use of herbs and, among these herbs, garlic stands supreme. Throughout medical history it has been acknowledged as a wonderful medicine. Some of the claims made in the scrolls and parchments of the great civilizations can only be described, by today's standards, as miraculous and yet within this maze of mythology and folklore lie many discoveries which even today are treated with respect. Indeed, so great is the current scientific interest in plant-based medicines that 'new' discoveries are being made, founded on hard medical facts. It is not surprising that garlic is being examined, along with many other herbs, in a very serious and scientific manner. Laboratories throughout the world are working to unlock the secrets held within the simple garlic corm.

It is said that there is nothing new under the sun and one can imagine the ancient doctors and philosophers such as Hippocrates and Aristotle, Galen and Celsus, sitting in the heavens with their respective gods, smiling down on the labours of our twentieth century medical research teams and saying 'but we told you that years ago'.

Garlic is a fascinating herb surrounded by folklore and yet still possessing remarkably effective powers, which are now becoming more widely accepted than they have been for the past 100 years. This then is the story of garlic and it is in many respects the story of herbal medicine. Within these pages we shall look at the history, examine the claims which are made and attempt to unravel the secrets contained in both the ancient writings and the most up-to-date scientific reports.

CHAPTER ONE

VICE AND VIRTUES

Anyone who knows anything at all about garlic is aware that it has a very pungent smell which leaves a disagreeable odour on the breath of those who eat it. Although this book is written to extol the virtues of garlic, it would be wrong to ignore what many people consider to be its only vice. Not that there is universal agreement that the smell and taste of garlic are unpleasant – in many countries of the world it is so popular and widely used that the inhabitants are unaware that it smells at all. In countries such as Italy and Russia and in many other nations throughout Europe and Asia, garlic is acceptable. It is only because in this country we have largely ignored and neglected the culinary properties of garlic that we notice the smell and condemn it as objectionable.

The smell which garlic leaves on the breath has also been responsible for its neglect by medical practitioners, particularly since it has been possible to replace them with synthetic drugs. This is most unfortunate since garlic certainly has a great ability to combat a host of diseases and conditions without having any side effects other than its smell. The odour of garlic has made it the target for jokes ever since the earliest literature. We can learn from the writings of the Greeks and Romans that although the common masses ate garlic with relish it was frowned upon by the nobility. Garlic eaters were prevented from entering some of the early Greek temples and the Romans banned them from the Senate.

The number of references to garlic in

literature testify not just to its smell but also to just how widespread was the use of the herb. It is mentioned in some of the great Greek tragedies, and Shakespeare uses it as a comic device in at least two of his plays.

PROTECTION AGAINST EVIL

It is almost certain that this unpleasant aspect of garlic gave rise to the many legends and superstitions that linked garlic with evil spirits. It was believed that the very smell of garlic would drive away devils, and in Central Europe it was a well known protection against vampires.

Garlic was never very popular amongst the English upper classes. Its smell was frowned upon and was much associated with the 'working classes'. In spite of this major disadvantage garlic still survived and enjoyed a tremendous reputation as a medicine and its use, as we shall see later, is recorded throughout history in the treatment of many ailments. It was one of the most effective and popular remedies that the herbalists had at their disposal and they made excellent use of it.

One of the strange things about garlic is that when it is freshly harvested the corm has virtually no odour attached to it. It is only when the cloves are bruised or cut that the characteristic odour is released. This is the result of an enzymatic action which takes place and converts one of the components in garlic into a substance called allicin. The allicin is contained in the essential oil of garlic and is responsible for its anti-bacterial and anti-inflammatory properties. We shall look more closely at the medicinal substances present in garlic corms in a later chapter and for the present it is sufficient to say that garlic's odour is an unavoidable property of the natural oil which is used for remedial purposes. Many people prefer to obtain their garlic by using garlic capsules (or perles as they are often called) so that the smell and taste are avoided.

OIL OF GARLIC

The essential oil of garlic is very strong and penetrating. One of the old folk remedies for whooping cough was to place slices of garlic corm in the shoes of the sufferer. On the face of it this seems a quite pointless and laughable method of treatment, but modern research into garlic tells us that within ten minutes of garlic oil being applied to the soles of the feet its smell can be detected on the breath.

The oil is so potent that even the most minute trace can be detected on the breath. It is so penetrating that there have been reports that when pregnant mothers have eaten garlic the smell can be passed through the womb to the breath of a new born baby. This fact was recorded in *Lancet* during 1973.

There have been many methods employed over the years to avoid the smell. Certain herbs when eaten with garlic will help to mask the odour; amongst the most popular of these is parsley. It seems probable that these other herbs do not kill the odoriferous substance but merely mask its odour by producing a flavour and aroma of their own.

Scientists are constantly looking for methods to produce a completely odourless garlic and have had some success in growing strains of garlic which have the same taste and properties but which have a lower level of odour. The Japanese in particular have been very active in trying to produce odourless garlic and one recently reported method was to boil garlic in honey to remove the smell.

ODOURLESS CAPSULES

For the last fifty years garlic oil has been available in the form of soft gelatine capsules. They are easy to swallow and pass through the stomach to the small intestine and the oil is then absorbed into the bloodstream. This method almost completely overcomes the odour problem and for many people it is a welcome alternative to eating the fresh corm. The great majority of those who take garlic capsules regularly report no detectable odour or taste, although it will tend not to pass unnoticed during the close contact of a kiss!

There are several brands of garlic capsules (often called perles) which are available at health food stores. The very fact that well in excess of one hundred million of these capsules are purchased in the United Kingdom every year does, I believe, indicate that the problem of odour is largely overcome through their use.

There are many specialist health food stores in all the major shopping centres throughout the country. These shops carry a wide range of foods and, in addition to herbal remedies, vitamin and mineral food supplements, they will certainly have in stock one or more types of garlic preparations, including garlic perles. Most good quality greengrocers and even some of the supermarket chains will stock fresh garlic corms which can be used in cooking.

Having dealt with garlic's vice, we can now begin to explore its many virtues. It is possible, with the preparation described above, to avoid the unpleasant social consequences that used to handicap garlic lovers, whilst still obtaining all the medicinal value of this most important herb.

Garlic can be treated as both food and medicine. As a food you will either like it or hate it, but as a medicine you certainly cannot ignore it. It is safe and effective over a wide range of conditions and, if taken in the correct dosage in the form of garlic perles, there is no need to be afraid of its single disadvantage.

THE PLANT – A DESCRIPTION

The Rodale Herb Book (Rodale Press, Emmaus, Pa, U.S.A.) describes garlic as 'a ruffian with a heart of gold', claiming that it has a 'wealth of talents' of value in the kitchen, the garden and the medicine chest. Garlic is undoubtedly one of the oldest and most versatile of all cultivated herbs. Its origin is uncertain but it is believed to have spread into Europe and the Middle East from somewhere in Central Asia. It belongs to the same group of plants as the onion, leek, chive and shallot and is a member of the lily family. It has always intrigued botanists that such a pungent smelling herb should be related to the symbol of purity. Its botanical name is *Allium sativum*; language experts believe that the 'al' comes from the Celtic word meaning 'burning' and 'sativum' means 'to cultivate'.

There are several varieties of garlic but it is the *Allium sativum* which is most often used in cooking and almost always in medicine. The plant consists of a bulb which sends up a few slender sprouts, the leaves grow to one or two feet in length and the flower is a cluster of tiny white blossoms. These, however, are rarely seen since the plant is harvested before the flowers appear. It is the bulb of the garlic which is used. The leaves themselves can be included in salads but they do not possess any of the medicinal properties of the bulb.

The bulb contains several smaller segments called cloves. A garlic bulb will normally contain eight to twelve of these cloves enclosed within a thin white or pinkish-white skin. They will grow in most climates, although for commercial cultivation they normally require a fairly lengthy, warm growing period. The garlic is a perennial plant and the dried corms can be saved and replanted to grow new plants in the same way that onions are grown.

There are three popular kinds which are normally grown. These are the common white, which has a white skin covering the clove, the pink garlic which can be harvested earlier than the white and a more red coloured plant which is a much slower grower although it does produce large cloves. There is also a wild garlic sometimes called Ramson which is not used very often as a food and hardly at all as a medicine. It does not have the clove formation in the bulb.

The member of the onion family which most closely resembles garlic is the shallot, which was brought to England by the Crusaders returning from the East during the Middle Ages. It has been regularly grown in this country since that time and is almost as strong smelling as the garlic. Most shallots are used for pickling.

The most widely eaten member of this family of plants is the onion which is so well known that there is no need for a description of it in this book. Onion and garlic contain many similar active principles which are used in medicine although the onion is not as powerful nor has it such a wide spectrum of use as the garlic. Other members in this group of plants are the chive, and the leek.

NUTRITIONAL CONTENT

It used to be thought that the value of garlic in medicine was based upon the action of the vitamins and minerals which it contains. In the late 1930s two American doctors suggested that, because of its high therapeutic action, garlic must contain large amount of vitamins. However, modern studies have disproved this theory and because it is eaten in relatively small quantities it does not provide a good nutritional source of vitamins unless large amounts are present in the diet. *The Handbook of the Nutritional Contents of Food*, prepared for the United States Department of Agriculture, gives the following information about the nutritional composition of garlic.

Proportions of Nutrients in Raw Garlic

Nutrient	Percentage content
Carbohydrate	31
Protein	6
Fat	0·2
Water	61

Mineral Content Per 100 Grams of Garlic

Mineral	Content
Calcium	29mg
Phosphorus	202mg
Iron	0·5mg
Sodium	19mg
Potassium	529mg

Vitamin Content Per 100 Grams of Raw Garlic

Vitamin	Content
A	trace
B_1 (thiamin)	0·25mg
B_2 (riboflavin)	0·08mg
Nicotinamide	0·5mg
C	15mg

These figures are supported by recently published Japanese Food Standard component analysis which give similar quantities although they are not identical. This is not surprising since the vitamin and mineral content of all natural products will vary depending upon the conditions which govern its growth i.e., type of soil, climate, time of harvesting, length of storage, etc. From these figures we can see that it is not a particularly rich source of any nutrient and is probably best thought of as a spice rather than a nutritious food.

None of the nutritional tables given make any reference to the relatively high sulphur content of garlic. Garlic contains more sulphur than onions or any of the other members of the family to which they belong and the allium family in general contains more sulphur than all other vegetables. This content of sulphur containing compounds is very important when we come to consider the medicinal composition of garlic later in the book.

REMEDIAL PROPERTIES

Although the total nutritional value of garlic is not great it does contain two other nutrients worthy of special consideration. These are a rare trace element called selenium and an unusual type of vitamin B_1.

Garlic contains more selenium than most other vegetables. Trace elements are essential to the correct functioning of the body, but the amounts used by the metabolism are so minute that they are often measured in micrograms. Selenium is becoming better known as more information becomes available about its action. It is the subject of a lot of attention by medical and nutritional research teams who are investigating its role as a very important trace element. Its activity is closely related to that of vitamin E in that it is an anti-oxidant and so helps to prevent pollution of the blood stream. It is thought that it can help prevent heavy metals such as mercury and lead from poisoning the body. The anti-oxidant properties of selenium may be one of the contributory factors in garlic's role in the prevention of heart attacks and normalizing blood pressure.

The chemical name for vitamin B_1 is thiamin and research workers in Japan have discovered a highly biologically active compound of vitamin B called allithiamin in garlic. Vitamin B_1 is not easy for the body to assimilate but when the special compound in garlic is present the vitamin B_1 is more quickly and efficiently absorbed, so much so that the level of vitamin B in the blood increases dramatically. This is important because vitamin B_1 plays a very important role in the body's metabolism, helping to keep the nerves healthy and preventing depression. Deficiency of vitamin B_1 leads to the disease known as beri-beri.

Another function of vitamin B_1 is that it assists the body to burn up carbohydrates to provide energy. If it is in short supply this process is interrupted and glucose is not properly utilized and is converted to fat. The results of vitamin B_1 deficiency are palpitations, muscular weakness and nerve troubles. As we shall read in a later chapter, the Greek athletes and Roman soldiers valued garlic because it gave them strength and energy, possibly because the allithiamin helped to convert the carbohydrate in their food into extra energy.

There are a great many separate nutrients and other substances to be found in garlic and its action cannot be explained by the presence of any single one. Like so many natural products the total effect is dependent on the *combined* action of the individual component parts. With the knowledge we now possess about the composition of garlic it is much easier to understand and explain the claims that are made for its healing powers.

CHAPTER TWO

THE HISTORICAL EVIDENCE

The historical fact that garlic has been used for many thousands of years as both food and medicine is indisputable. The ancient records show that for over 5,000 years garlic's healing powers have been used to treat a wide spectrum of disease. It is mentioned in the Old Testament, in the great writings of the Greeks, by Babylonians, Chinese, Romans and Egyptians. The Vikings took garlic with them on their long sea voyages. From the early healers and philosophers such as Galen, Hippocrates and Pliny, throughout the Middle Ages, in an unbroken chain to some of the great modern healers such as Schweitzer and Bircher-Benner, we can follow the story of garlic. From the building of the pyramids to the terrible world wars of our present century we can see the healing power of garlic at work.

EARLY RECORDS

We do not know when garlic was first used as a food or a medicine. It is believed that the very earliest references can be traced to Babylon. The Chinese have certainly been known to use it as a medicine since 2000 B.C. and ancient Egyptian history records its existence in an inscription found in a pyramid reputed to have been built almost 5,000 years ago. In fact some garlic corms were found within the tomb of Tutankhamen. The bible confirms that garlic was highly thought of as a food by the early Israelite slaves who built the great pyramids. It was reputed to give them strength and nourishment.

The Ancient Chinese

The tradition of herbal medicine in China is maintained until today. The Chinese call the garlic herb *suan*. The story of how the followers of Emperor Huang-ti were climbing a mountain and ate a poisonous plant and became very ill is recorded in the *Calendar of the Hsia*. This book, written 4,000 years ago, tells how their lives were saved by eating the wild garlic which grew locally. From that time until today, garlic has been extensively used by Chinese physicians.

The Ancient Hebrews

In the Bible (Numbers 11:5) we read that, as Moses led the Israelites through the wilderness, amongst the things they missed most was garlic. The Jews were great believers in garlic, they cultivated it along with leeks and onions as a staple part of their diet but to them, as to many other races, it was more than just a food, it was a potent medicine of such power that it was ascribed magical properties.

In the Middle Ages Jewish superstition suggested that the carrying of garlic corms about the person would protect one from the infectious diseases which decimated whole populations in medieval Europe.

They could only account for its effectiveness by ascribing to it the power of appeasing the evil spirits which brought the disease. Today we know that garlic is an effective natural antibiotic capable of combating bacteria.

Garlic in Islam

Among other great religions of the world we can also find references to garlic. It is mentioned in the Koran and according to ancient tradition when Satan stepped out of the Garden of Eden after Adam had taken that fateful bite of the apple, garlic sprang up from the place where his left foot fell and onion from his right foot.

The Ancient Egyptians

It is interesting to trace some of the ancient methods of practising medicine to see how science has developed over the years. It is widely accepted that the Egyptians were the first civilization to really practise medicine. They had developed a comprehensive system of training through the priests who were the official medical practitioners of the day and were subject to formal education and examination.

In Europe it was the monks who copied out by hand the old textbooks on herbal medicine and it often happened that the centre of their religious life, the monastery, was also the ancient equivalent of a hospital. Many of the medicinal recipes they used had been handed down from the earliest Greek and Egyptian texts and among the conditions they treated with garlic were worms, headaches, heart problems, asthma and problems of menstruation, plus of course coughs and colds.

Medical historians sometimes compare the knowledge of these early Egyptian physicians with that of the European herbalists in the Middle Ages. They find that little changed and that the traditional remedies such as garlic had stood the test of time. These early healers knew that they had a powerful medicine which could kill the cause of many diseases. We now know that the properties which have led garlic to be dubbed 'Russian Penicillin' are not miraculous powers at all but that garlic does in fact have antibiotic properties which can cure disease.

STRENGTH AND ENDURANCE

We have already seen how during the construction of the pyramids of Cheops, the workers went on strike because they were deprived of garlic. They felt that it was essential to give them strength and endurance. G. J. Binding in his book *About Garlic* (Thorsons, Wellingborough, Northants) tells us how the onion and garlic are still widely cultivated in Egypt today. He believes that the strength and endurance displayed by Egyptians in many sports demanding great physical powers, such as weight lifting or cross-channel swimming, can be ascribed to the use of garlic.

Garlic is also reputed to have been used by the Greek athletes, who ate it to prepare themselves for their feats of strength and endurance during the original Olympic Games. A far cry from the reported use of drugs and steroids by their modern counterparts. They also fed it to their warriors to give them confidence before going into battle.

Many modern herbalists would testify to the tonic properties of garlic and so these ancient beliefs were perhaps not without foundation after all. But the Greeks did not just use garlic for its strength-giving properties or as a food; for them it was as much a medicine as any other plant or herb they knew.

EARLY GREEK MEDICINE

Today medical doctors still take the Hippocratic Oath, based on the tradition of medicine founded by Hippocrates. Hippocrates used garlic for a variety of diseases as well as using it to treat wounds, leprosy and toothache. He also recommends it as a laxative and diuretic.

Important though Hippocrates was, it was another Greek who made what is possibly the greatest contribution to the practice of herbal medicine. Dioscorides was chief doctor to the Roman army. His herbal books formed the basis of herbal medicine until the end of the Middle Ages. As he travelled with the armies he was able to accumulate local knowledge from the countries he visited. It was not so much the recipes which he compounded that give his work importance, but rather the precision with which he recorded the details of weights, dosages and methods of preparation of his medicines. These were closely followed by generations of medical herbalists. Dioscorides' careful study and recording of the plant kingdom completely changed the way in which herbalists thought about plants, and herbal medicine owes him a great debt.

Lloyd J. Harris in *The Book of Garlic* (Panjandrum/ Aris Books, Los Angeles) includes the following quotation from the Greek herbal of Dioscorides, translated by J. Berendes. Talking about garlic he relates the following:

It is sharp, biting, wind-producing, excites the belly, dries out the stomach, creates thirst and reduces growths on the body skin. If eaten it helps to eliminate tapeworm, it drives out the urine. It is good against snake bite with wine or when crushed in wine. It is good against the bite of a rabid dog. It makes the voice clear and soothes continuous coughing when eaten raw or boiled. Boiled with oregano, it kills lice and bed bugs. It doth clear the arteries. Burnt and mixed with honey, it heals white skin spots, herpetic eruptions, liver spots, leprosy and scurvy. Boiled with pine wood and incense, it soothes toothache when the solution is kept in the mouth. Garlic plus fig leaves and cumin is a plaster against the bite of the shrew mouse. Boiling the umbel flower is good for a sitzbath (sitting bath) to help the coming of menstruation and placenta. For the same purpose it can be smoked. A mush from garlic and black olives is a diuretic. It is helpful in dropsy.

An impressive list, especially when, as we shall discover later, many of these uses have now been proved to have a sound, scientific base. Dioscorides often compounded garlic with other ingredients and used medicines to treat many disorders including skin diseases, worms, coughs, bites and stings, asthma and the arterial problems. Many of these uses are still practised by modern herbalists, particularly in the treatment of coughs, colds and other bronchial problems, wounds, bites and stings. The Greeks used raw garlic mixed with wine, honey and other ingredients. Their successors, however, recommend garlic in capsule form as this is far more convenient and less objectionable.

GARLIC IN THE ROMAN WORLD

That other great Mediterranean power, the Roman Empire, also held garlic in high esteem. They too enjoyed it as a food and fed it in large amounts to their soldiers for strength and courage as well as health. Indeed, Roman legions carried garlic with them on their many campaigns and were responsible for introducing it to many countries they conquered. The humble Roman citizen enjoyed his garlic but the aristocracy frowned upon the smell which was distasteful to them. It was renowned as an aphrodisiac and mixed with other herbs into potent 'love potions'. Virgil, the poet, also mentions garlic and tells us that it was essential to maintain the strength of the farm workers as they gathered the harvest.

Possibly the most famous of the Roman physicians was Galen whose teachings influenced medical thought and practice for a thousand years. He gave his name to the term 'galenical' which refers to remedies of vegetable, not synthetic origin. The word is still in common use among herbalists. He is also credited with having christened garlic 'The Poor Man's Treacle'. He spoke and taught many pupils about garlic's healing powers and recommended it highly as an antidote against poisons. Today we would refer to them as toxins of the blood, but the principle still holds good and garlic stands supreme after thousands of years of use.

The most prolific supporter of garlic in the Roman world of medicine was Pliny, a famous naturalist who, in his 'Natural History', gives very many uses for the herb. Herbalists are still using garlic to treat many of the conditions encountered by Pliny and his contemporaries: respiratory infections, wounds, gastro-intestinal disorders all respond to garlic's healing powers.

CHINESE HERBAL MEDICINE

The Chinese are another race who value garlic as a medicine and make use of its properties to treat a whole range of illness from high blood pressure through to gastro-intestinal problems. The use of wild garlic in China was first recorded in 2000 B.C. and it was probably two thousand years later that garlic was first cultivated in Central Asia from where it found its way east to China. It was used to preserve meat, and food technologists have recently shown that the effect of garlic on certain microbes can help to preserve and extend the freshness and keeping properties of canned meats. Here again is an illustration of a use for garlic, practised over many centuries, being proved by modern scientific research.

The many uses to which garlic is used in

Chinese herbal medicine make it almost a panacea – a cure-all. It is claimed that because of its wide activity it can help in conditions of asthma, bronchitis and colds, to clear poisons from the body, to heal abscesses, wounds and many other problems. Indeed, some Chinese herbalists claim that they have cured tuberculosis with garlic, used as an inhalant and taken internally. Reports from India also suggest its use for the same disease. There is still a very strong tradition of herbal medicine in China and the use of garlic by the modern herbal practitioners will be dealt with in a later chapter.

As I have just said, India is another country where garlic has been used for hundreds of years and where it is still used today for the treatment of many diseases. In the early writings of ancient India there are many references to it as a food and a medicinal herb.

GROWTH OF KNOWLEDGE

From these early civilizations the use of garlic has been passed on and has continued to the present day. Following the collapse of the Roman Empire few new references to the use of garlic appear and it is not until the Middle Ages that we again begin to read of its medicinal use. Once the printing press had been invented and a great many books became available and were read by many more people, knowledge once again began to expand. The early herbalists undoubtedly relied upon folklore and this knowledge about herbs was passed down from generation to generation by word of mouth. They discovered new uses and were able, very slowly, by observation and experiment, to produce a new philosophy of herbalism. In very broad terms this can be summed up in the following short statement: for every ailment, nature provides a cure. Written works of the early herbal experts documented the known uses of various plants and are referred to as 'herbals'. The most famous and widely read of the English herbalists was Nicholas Culpeper (1616–1654) and *Culpeper's Complete Herbal* is still in print today.

DOCTRINE OF SIGNATURES

One of the popular herbal theories of the late Middle Ages is the Doctrine of Signatures. This suggests that by examining the physical characteristics of plants man may read how nature intended them to be used for health. Therefore it was believed that because the garlic plant had a hollow stem it would be of benefit in afflictions of the windpipe, hence its use in all types of respiratory disorders such as coughs, colds catarrh, asthma and bronchial problems. These theories are now, of course, just a part of herbal history and cannot stand the critical examination of modern science, however the principle still remains true that garlic has many uses which have remained unchanged, even though our knowledge of the herb itself has considerably expanded. Today we do not have to rely on faith and superstition; we have a mass of facts which *prove* garlic's effectiveness.

THE OLD HERBALS

It is interesting to look at some of the old herbals to see what they can teach us about the use of garlic. Culpeper died in 1654 and the following extract is from an old edition of his *English Physician and Complete Herbal*, published in 1813.

CULPEPER's
ENGLISH PHYSICIAN;

AND COMPLETE

HERBAL.

TO WHICH ARE NOW FIRST ADDED,

Upwards of One Hundred Additional HERBS,

WITH A DISPLAY OF THEIR

MEDICINAL AND OCCULT PROPERTIES,

PHYSICALLY APPLIED TO

The CURE of all DISORDERS incident to MANKIND.

TO WHICH ARE ANNEXED,

RULES for compounding MEDICINE according to the true SYSTEM of NATURE;

FORMING A COMPLETE

FAMILY DISPENSATORY,

And Natural SYSTEM of PHYSIC,

BEAUTIFIED AND ENRICHED WITH

ENGRAVINGS of upwards of Four Hundred and Fifty different PLANTS, And a SET of ANATOMICAL FIGURES.

ILLUSTRATED WITH NOTES AND OBSERVATIONS,
CRITICAL AND EXPLANATORY;

By the late E. SIBLY, M. D. Fellow of the Harmonic Philosophical Society at PARIS;
and Author of the Complete ILLUSTRATION of ASTROLOGY.

VOL. I. Containing the HERBAL.

FIFTEENTH EDITION, improved by the Addition of the LINNÆAN NAME to each Herb, Plant, and Tree;
and a LIFE of CULPEPER.

LONDON:

PRINTED BY W. LEWIS, ST. JOHN'S SQUARE, FOR THE PROPRIETOR; AND SOLD
AT THE ENCYCLOPÆDIA OFFICE, 17, AVE-MARIA-LANE; AND BY ALL
BOOKSELLERS IN TOWN AND COUNTRY.

M.DCCC.XIII.

Figure 1. Title page of Culpeper's *English Physician and Complete Herbal.*

GARLIC. Allium.

IT is fo univerfally known, that I fhall decline troubling my readers with any defcription of it.

Government and Virtues. Mars owns this herb. It provoketh urine and women's courfes, and helpeth the biting of mad dogs and other venomous creatures; it killeth worms in children, cutteth and bringeth forth tough phlegm, purgeth the head, helpeth the lethargy, and is a good prefervative againft, and a remedy for, any plague-fore, or foul ulcer; it taketh away fpots and blemifhes of the fkin; eafeth pains of the ears, and ripeneth and breaketh impofthumes and other fwellings. It has been noticed that onions are equally effectual for the faid purpofes, but garlic hath many peculiar virtues which the onion cannot boaft of: for inftance, it hath a fpecial quality to remove all inconveniences proceeding from corrupt agues or mineral vapours, or from drinking ftagnated or unclean water; as alfo by taking of wolf-bane, hen-bane, hemlock, or other poifonous herbs. It is alfo exceeding good in hydropic difeafes, the jaundice, falling ficknefs, cramps, convulfions, the piles or hemorrhoids, and other cold difeafes. However, having fhowed its many virtues, it is alfo neceffary that its vices fhould not be concealed: its heat is very vehement, and every thing of that defcription naturally conveys ill vapours to the brain; in choleric cafes it adds fuel to the fire; in men oppreffed with melancholy, it extenuates the humour, and confounds the idea with ftrange vifions and fancies; and therefore ought to be taken with the ftricteft care by thofe whofe ill difpofition of body will not admit of a liberal application. A few cummin-feeds, or a green bean or two, being chewed after eating garlic, will entirely remove the difagreeable fmell of the breath proceeding therefrom.

Figure 2. Section on garlic in Culpeper's herbal.

It is interesting to note that in Culpeper's time the garlic was so well known that he did not feel it necessary to trouble his readers by describing the plant. Culpeper too was conscious of the disadvantage of garlic's characteristic odour on the breath and felt it necessary to advise his readers that by eating a few cummin seeds or a few green beans after the garlic, then the disagreeable smell would be removed. We read how in the seventeenth century the traditional use of garlic was much the same as that practised by the Egyptians, Romans and Greeks.

It seems strange to read that a herb such as garlic could be thought to be ruled by the planet Mars. This is a reference to the old belief, which probably started in Babylon but was developed by the Greeks, that the sun, moon, planets and constellations of the zodiac ruled not only people but also plants. The planet of Mars, the God of War, ruled plants with thorns or very strong taste (like garlic). They were also governed by the zodiac sign of Aries. Obviously it was not a belief based on scientific fact. Even so, it is a constant source of amazement that whatever the method of deciding to employ garlic or however its usage was shrouded in mystery the fact remains that these primitive doctors knew which herb to use for the best effect.

Many herbals similar to Culpeper's were published and were widely read, much to the consternation of the medical profession who had jealously guarded their secrets which could now be read by anyone able to understand. Among the most widely read were *Parkinson's Herbal,* Sir John Hill's *Family Herbal* and Dr Fernie's *Herbal Simples*. They all included sections on garlic's powerful role in medicine.

In *The Herb Book* by John Lust (Benedict Lust Publications, New York) there is a list of garlic's many traditional uses and properties. It is labelled an anthelmintic, antispasmodic, carminative, chologogue, digestive, diuretic, expectorant and febrifuge. These and other herbal terms are explained in the Appendix at the back of this book.

GARLIC AND PLAGUES

It is not only in the English herbal tradition that garlic is prominent. In France, where it is so highly valued as a food, there are a few references to its use in medicine. In fact one of the most famous of all the legends about garlic is concerned with a terrible plague which occurred in the south of France in the eighteenth century. Thousands of people were dying and it became a problem to find someone prepared to bury the corpses. Four convicts under sentence of death were released from prison against an undertaking that they would carry out the burials of the victims. No one could explain how these thieves remained immune to the plague when they were continually exposed to it. Finally they released their secret which was that every day they drank garlic macerated in wine, to protect them from disease. This mixture became known as Four Thieves Vinegar and I am informed that it is still drunk today.

There were many plagues during the Middle Ages and England did not escape. There is a Tudor House in Chester which, during the Great Plague of 1665 housed a family who escaped the consequences of the plague even though many thousands were dying. The legend has it that the cellars of this building were full of garlic and it is this which protected the entire occupants of the house from the effects of the plague, whilst their neighbours were dying about them.

Such stories are common in Europe. How much of it is fact and how much part of folklore we shall never know. We do know that garlic was used to disinfect burial grounds to keep the plagues from spreading and of course our modern knowledge helps us to appreciate the properties of garlic which were likely to have been responsible for this protective action. The Spaniards are believed to have been responsible for introducing garlic to the American continent. Lloyd J. Harris in his *Book of Garlic* tells us how in the Santa Fe area it was used to cure horses with swollen necks and dogs from rabies and worms. They also used it for pains in the bowels in humans and to relieve flatulence. Among the American Indians there was a strong tradition of herbal medicine and garlic was used to relieve ear ache, stomach troubles, injuries to the foot and diphtheria.

MODERN APPROACHES

However, science was progressing and it became possible to synthesize drugs which began to replace herbs. By the beginning of the present century, the use of herbs had declined and the profession of herbalism was practised by fewer people. During the last hundred years garlic has not been a very popular remedy and is hardly ever prescribed by conventional medical doctors. Fortunately, however, there are signs that the interest in herbal medicine is reviving and with the current research work that is being undertaken, more and more people are returning to these well tried and trusted remedies which are free from side effects. Amongst them garlic has no equal.

Today we place more emphasis on preventative medicine than did our fore-fathers. Perhaps because garlic was a regular part of the diet of most races it was not necessary for the herbalist of the day to have to recommend it as a preventative medicine. The regular use of garlic does however help prevent a great many ills, especially the common winter ailments such as colds and flu. For fifty years, since the studies of the German physician Johan Höfels, garlic has been produced in gelatine capsules. This method of taking garlic has overcome the prejudice of many people to the herb's smell and taste. Capsules contain pure oil of garlic and are easy to swallow and do not have the unpleasant smell of raw garlic. All health food stores sell several brands and over 100,000,000 capsules are sold in the United Kingdom every year.

CHAPTER THREE

GARLIC IN THE KITCHEN AND GARDEN

Garlic is a member of the same family of plants as onions, yet whilst most kitchen gardens contain onions, leeks, shallots or chives, the garlic is much less popular, although it is not too difficult to cultivate in the British Isles. It is worthwhile planting some cloves both to ensure a fresh supply of fresh garlic and for general interest and novelty. Like the onion, it is not a very decorative plant and the best and most valuable part lies underground.

GROWING YOUR OWN

Garlic enjoys a light sandy soil which drains well and has a long growing season, ideally with lots of sunshine. The conditions mean that it is not a very practical proposition to grow it as a commercial crop but for the amateur gardener it is relatively easy to grow and requires little experience. Garlic grows very easily in the warm climate of Southern Europe and can be grown very cheaply. This makes it an uneconomical proposition for market gardeners in Britain although in Essex at least one producer plants five acres of garlic as a commercial crop with great success.

Method

No fresh manure other than bone meal is needed and the ideal soil is one that is free from clay and has been previously manured for another crop. It is best and safest to grow garlic from the corm (Thompson and Morgan of Ipswich can supply several different and interesting varieties) and the common corms can easily be purchased from a greengrocer. Remove the outer skin from the bulb to reveal clusters of tiny corms and carefully separate the corms being careful not to bruise them and plant in drills about $\frac{1}{2}$ in (1 cm) deep. Allow about 8 ins (20 cm) between the plants and 12 ins (30 cms) between rows.

In the warmer south-west planting can be done in November but for most of the country it is best to leave planting until March. Water at least once a week in dry weather and ensure good drainage. Garlic planted in March should be ready to harvest in October or November. Gather the bulbs when the leaves have withered and died away. *The Rodale Herb Book* recommends bending the stalks to the ground in late summer as a method of encouraging early ripening and, of course, the plants should not be allowed to flower.

Drying

Once gathered they should be allowed to dry out, away from direct sunlight. The best method is to remove most of the leaves and then hang the bulbs in bunches, *The Rodale Herb Book* also suggests storing them in net bags or old nylon stockings. Once dried, garlic will keep until required for use. Usually only the corms are used but if you are growing your own then a few fresh green leaves, finely chopped, make a tasty addition to a salad, or as a garnish.

Garlic only begins to give off its characteristic odour when it is cut or bruised. It is important at all stages to ensure that the bulbs are treated very gently to avoid bruising.

Growing Indoors

If you do not have a garden you may still like to try growing garlic indoors. Plant a clove in a plant pot filled with rich potting compost, keep out of direct sunlight until the shoot starts to show through, this should take approximately two to three weeks in a fairly cool place. Once the shoot is 2 ins (5 cm) long stand in the window and keep well watered.

ORGANIC GARDENING

There is an old agricultural technique which has been used by organic gardeners throughout the world for many years which is based on the idea that some plants will deter pests which are attracted to others. Therefore the plants which have a deterrent effect are planted amongst those which are subject to attack. Amongst these repellant plants garlic is well known to be a very effective pest controller. It takes up very little room in the garden, is extremely powerful and, at the same time, it is an easy plant to grow and has both culinary and medicinal uses. It is not a particularly decorative garden plant, but this will not deter the gardener who is determined to control pests without resorting to the use of chemicals. It is well understood that many pests thrive when crops are segregated, as in mass farming techniques, and by mixing garlic in with some of your more susceptible plants, effective pest control can be achieved without resort to artificial aids. Garlic has been known as a pesticide since the very earliest civilizations practised farming; it will not taint other crops although it is most successful with root crops. Because the odour of garlic is mainly confined within the bulb which is beneath the soil, there is no noticeable garlic smell in the garden.

Garlic can be planted beneath fruit trees, near cabbages and among the beans. If a row of garlic is planted between the rows of beans, it takes up very little room and is most successful in keeping away many varieties of pests. Roses, tomatoes, potatoes and peas are often very vulnerable to attack by common garden pests and much of the damage caused by insect infestation can be prevented by planting a few garlic corms near your plants. Other members of the garlic family such as chives, leeks and shallots can also be used, but with less effect. Garlic can also be planted near soft fruits such as raspberries with equally good results.

AS AN INSECTICIDE

Garlic is useful as an insecticide not just when planted but also when made into a spray which can be used on nearly all plants. One simple method is to soak crushed garlic corms in large vats of water and then spray on the plants which are at risk. David Greenstock who was connected with the Henry Doubleday Research Association, a well known organization in organic gardening circles, produced one method. Details of a do-it-yourself recipe are given in *The Rodale Herb Book*, based on Mr Greenstock's work. This involves soaking approximately 3 oz (75g) chopped garlic corms in about 2 fl oz (50ml) of mineral oil (i.e. liquid paraffin) for about 24 hours. This is then slowly mixed with one pint (575ml) of water in which $\frac{3}{4}$ oz (20g) of soap has been dissolved. Stir well and strain through muslin or old nylon stocking, then store in an earthenware or glass (not metal) container. It can be used diluted from one part to twenty parts of water, down to one part per hundred and is reputed to be effective against most common garden pests.

In the early 1970s reports appeared in the American press about garlic's effectiveness as a pesticide. Researchers at the University of California reported that even low concentrations of crude garlic extract could kill at least five species of mosquito larvae. Further experiments with a more refined extract gave even better results. The mosquito not only affects plants but also carries diseases such as yellow fever, malaria and encephalitis and the normal method of controlling them was to spray crops with a strong pesticide such as D.D.T. I think that D.D.T. is now banned by most countries, because not only does it kill insects, it also affects and can kill humans. How much safer it would have been for human life and the environment in general had a natural pesticide such as garlic been used in its place. It is perhaps unrealistic to expect that mass farming methods would be likely to accept a simple solution such as growing garlic and using it on a vast scale, but it does not preclude the amateur gardener from using these safe and effective methods.

Another interesting fact is that while insecticides kill many harmless insects and beetles that live alongside the dangerous pests, garlic does not. Many insects do have a vital role to play in the natural life cycle of our planet and especially the growth of healthy, abundant crops. The use of garlic is to be encouraged by all who are concerned about the environment and who want to follow a natural course of living. Garlic solutions have been shown to be effective in controlling a very wide range of pests including the various forms of mosquito already mentioned, plus onion fly, larvae, cabbage white caterpillar, pea weevil, cockroaches and many other common garden pests.

COOKING WITH GARLIC

I am sure that it will come as no surprise that the culinary history of this incredible herb is almost as ancient and as well documented as its medical history. It is mentioned in Chinese literature written 2,500 years ago and was used throughout the Orient and the Middle East. In countries around the Baltic and the Mediterranean there is a long history of the use of garlic in the kitchen. This tradition has, of course, continued into the modern era and garlic is found in many traditional recipes of all the cultures of the world. Some nations are renowned for their art in the skills of cookery. The French and the Chinese have long been regarded as masters in the art of producing appetizing dishes of delicate aroma and delicious taste. It is not by accident that garlic is exploited by French and Chinese chefs in the creation of some of their greatest dishes. Of course, because garlic is such a pungent herb it can completely dominate the flavour of a dish unless it is handled with great care. The skill of cooking with garlic is to bring out just the right amount of flavour, making the dish more appetizing and delicious without masking the flavour of the other ingredients.

Objections

Garlic certainly does not deserve the unsavoury reputation it seems to have acquired in Britain and America. Many of those who object to the use of garlic in cooking do so from prejudice rather than experience. They imagine that the herb is going to taint their breath and that it will make the whole meal unpleasant. Some even believe that because it is a hot and spicy herb it is indigestible. But garlic is a very valuable food which helps to promote the digestive processes.

Without wanting to detract in any way from the value of garlic as an ingredient in food it is only fair to state that it is doubtful whether most of us would be prepared to eat sufficient garlic as a regular thing, to provide enough for the medicinal purposes for which garlic is used. For the medicinal value to be effective it is necessary to have a regular daily dose and so the use of garlic capsules as a supplement or treatment rather than fresh garlic as a food, is the easiest and most convenient method. The capsules are easy to swallow and because they dissolve in the small intestine the effect on the breath is minimal. It is also much easier to ensure a correct dosage of the volatile oil by this method. Fortunately the garlic oil which contains the beneficial medicinal properties is not destroyed by heat and therefore the use of garlic in cooking does not prevent the medicinal benefits being obtained, but, as I have said, with capsules it is much easier to achieve the correct dose every day.

There are many surprises in store for the cook and the beneficiaries of her labours when she begins to experiment with garlic. This is not intended to be a cookery book but any introduction to garlic would be incomplete without some hints on its use and preparation in the kitchen. Also included are a few of the traditional recipes used throughout the world.

Smell

Before we start to cook with garlic a further word about its smell. Assuming that you enjoy the taste, there are one or two tips which have been passed down through the years to help eliminate some of the odour. The most popular of these is to include parsley when preparing a dish with garlic, either as a garnish or an ingredient. Parsley is a herb which is rich in chlorophyll, nature's deodorant and breath freshener, and this will help to clear the breath. Another antidote to the smell of garlic is milk and yet another is to drink water containing honey and a teaspoonful of lemon juice. I mention these tips for the newcomer to garlic, those who already know and appreciate its flavour will have found out for themselves that the misgivings of the uninitiated will soon be dispelled. Hopefully, as you begin to appreciate the flavour of garlic, the problem of its odour will not assume such a significance as it does when first introduced to the herb. Careful preparation and gentle handling is the secret.

Introducing Garlic

Nearly every book which introduces the reader to cooking with garlic begins with the basic method that has served so many others so well, it is the first step in acquiring the garlic habit. Cut a clove of garlic in half and rub it around the inside of the salad bowl, saucepan or other utensil in which the dish is to be prepared. This imparts a trace of the flavour of garlic to the salad or other dish and because it is such a gentle introduction most people find it perfectly acceptable. Of course, as you progress in your experiments you will want to add more and more garlic as you and your family acquire the taste.

There are an enormous number of methods of using garlic, it can be pressed, sliced, diced, minced or left whole. It can be boiled, fried, roasted and eaten raw. We have read earlier in this book how the odour of garlic is caused by an enzymatic process taking place, this only occurs when the corm is cut or bruised and therefore when garlic is cooked whole it has a very mild flavour. To prepare whole garlic cloves it is necessary to gently remove the outer skin. A favourite method of eating garlic is to slice it thinly and then fry it in vegetable oil until golden brown, serve it as you would fried onions.

Small containers of garlic powder can be purchased from your health food shop and this can be added to a number of dishes such as soups and casseroles in the same way you would use any other seasoning. The powder can also be mixed with table salt and sprinkled as usual. Most soups will be improved if a clove of garlic is finely chopped and added to the pan with the other ingredients. As with any method of introducing garlic it is better to start with a little and gradually increase the amount as you acquire the taste. Generally speaking it is true that the rougher the treatment you hand out to your garlic, the stronger will be its flavour. Conversely, if you treat it gently the flavour and aroma will be more delicate.

Here are a few traditional garlic dishes collected from various countries, you may like to try some of them yourself. Your favourite recipe book will almost certainly include others which use garlic and, by trial and error you will discover the method and quantity best suited to your taste.

RECIPES

Garlic Butter

This traditional French method of flavouring butter with garlic is to peel and chop the garlic cloves very fine. They are then pounded into the butter. One small clove to 8 oz (200g) butter is probably enough to begin with but you will want to add more as you acquire the taste.

Vegetable Soup
1½ pints (850ml) stock
2 medium-sized carrots
1 onion
1 turnip
1 large tomato
1 large potato
3 cloves garlic
celery
salt and pepper

Place the stock in a large saucepan. Grate the turnip, carrot, potato and celery, slice the peeled tomato and chop the onion and garlic very fine. Add all the vegetables to the pan. Bring to the boil and hold for two or three minutes whilst removing any scum. Cover and simmer for two hours. Season to taste.

Herb Bread
Prepare garlic butter as above. Slice a French loaf and spread the garlic butter onto each slice adding a light sprinkling of herbs to each slice. Gather the slices back into the loaf shape and wrap with silver foil. Place in oven at 425°F / 215°C (Gas Mark 7) and heat for 30 minutes. Serve hot with soup. Alternatively garlic butter can be spread on hot toast.

Mushroom Salad
8 oz (225g) mushrooms
1 clove garlic
Lemon juice
Vegetable oil (olive, sunflower)
Parsley
Salt and pepper

Wash and trim the mushrooms; cut into very thin slices. Cut the clove of garlic in half and rub it around the inside of the salad bowl. Discard the garlic, it has already introduced the flavour to the dish. Place the mushrooms in the bowl and pour 3 or 4 tablespoonsful of oil and the juice of $\frac{1}{2}$ a lemon over them. Season lightly with salt and pepper and sprinkle with parsley.

Serves 4. Serve with green salad, cold meat or as an *hors d'oeuvre*.

Mediterranean Roast Lamb
Shoulder of lamb
3 cloves garlic
3 pieces of fresh rosemary or dried rosemary leaves
Vegetable oil
6 oz (175g) stock
Salt and pepper

Make 6 deep cuts in the joint with a sharp knife. Peel garlic and cut in half. Press a piece of garlic and rosemary into each cut. Brush the meat with vegetable oil and season. Wrap joint in foil. Allow 30 minutes per 1 lb (450g) weight of meat plus 30 minutes and cook in oven at 375°F/190°C (Gas Mark 5) for half the cooking time. Unwrap foil and continue cooking so that the meat browns. 15 minutes before end of cooking pour on stock. Use stock to make a gravy.

Aïoli Sauce
(A traditional garlic sauce from Provence.)
4 large garlic cloves
1 egg yolk
1 cupful salad oil
Salt

Peel the garlic and chop finely. Place in dish and mash with egg yolk, using a mortar if available or, alternatively, the handle of a heavy knife. When well mashed, add salt to season. When finely ground add the oil a drop at a time. Continue to mix as you add the oil.

Aïoli sauce is used as you would mayonnaise.

CHAPTER FOUR

MODERN HERBAL USAGE

We have read in earlier chapters how garlic has a long and distinguished history which continues in an unbroken chain since the earliest civilizations. There is undoubtedly a lot that we can learn from the historical background to this medicinal plant but, although this is extremely important, it would be wrong to leave the reader with the impression that garlic is just an old-fashioned remedy. There exists today a very strong herbal tradition which is backed up by modern medical research facilities and, in the case of garlic, this is leading to a renewed interest and a continuing and developing use of its medicinal properties. Throughout the East, and particularly in the Indian subcontinent, the use of garlic is as widespread as it has ever been and nowhere is this more true than in China. Chinese herbal medicine makes extensive use of many of the traditional herbs and, according to Chinese herbalists, if you have garlic in your kitchen you possess something very close to a panacea. It can be used to treat a wide range of conditions including asthma, bronchitis, colds, diarrhoea, worms, abscesses, and many more. It is claimed that the garlic acts as an antibiotic, effective against a wide range of bacteria without having any side effects and that it also possesses many other virtues which make it the supreme treatment for many disorders.

RESPIRATORY TROUBLES
Chinese herbal medicine contains numerous

references to treatments for colds, coughs, asthma, bronchitis and other conditions of the respiratory tract. Recipes exist for the juice of garlic mixed with honey and other, stronger garlic syrups which are recommended for colds, coughs, sore throats, hoarseness, loss of voice, asthma and bronchitis. Richard Lucas, in his absorbing book *Secrets of the Chinese Herbalists* (Thorsons, Wellingborough, Northants) gives a recipe for a garlic syrup which is made by pouring a pint (575ml) of boiling water over 2 oz (50g) of finely chopped garlic; this is allowed to stand for ten hours in a closed container. It is then strained and a tablespoonful of vinegar is added, enough honey is then added to this mixture to form a syrup. This syrup is claimed to have expectorant properties for such problems as dry, hacking coughs and chronic bronchitis.

Chopped garlic in boiling water with a little vinegar added also makes an excellent inhalant. It is mixed in a bowl and the head is then covered with a towel and the vapours inhaled to clear nasal congestion. As I have said, in Europe in the Middle Ages garlic was used as one of the most effective preventatives known, against the various plagues which devastated whole populations. The Chinese healers similarly believed strongly in the preventative role of garlic. There is also a lot of evidence in Chinese literature for the use of garlic in the treatment of tuberculosis. Although this condition is so serious that it is essential that any treatment must be conducted under expert medical supervision, it is interesting to note that there are grounds for believing that garlic can be of help even in such a serious disease.

INTESTINAL DISORDERS

The Chinese also use garlic in the treatment of many ailments of the bowels. Problems such as colitis, diarrhoea, dysentery and many other intestinal upsets can be safely and successfully treated with garlic and either the fresh garlic clove or garlic capsules may be used. One garlic capsule taken three times a day is usually enough to correct mild cases of diarrhoea or dysentery and for more persistent cases up to six capsules a day can be taken. Garlic has the ability to destroy harmful bacteria in the intestines without affecting the beneficial organisms which aid digestion. In fact, it is believed by many that it has a *positive* benefit on the intestinal bacteria.

While the beneficial intestinal bacteria aid the digestion of food and play an important role in the synthesis (or production) of some of the B group vitamins, the harmful bacteria have a toxic effect resulting in putrefaction which can cause diarrhoea, dysentery and other intestinal disorders. Experiments have shown very clearly that while garlic has the power to destroy the harmful bacteria, it encourages the growth of the beneficial, without any side effects. These properties are used by herbalists throughout the world and western research has confirmed the findings of the ancient Chinese herbalists.

One of the health hazards encountered by many British people who travel abroad on holiday or business is that the change of climate, diet and water often leads to gastro-intestinal disturbances causing sickness or diarrhoea. Many of these problems can be avoided if garlic capsules are taken regularly for two weeks before going abroad and the use continued during the time spent away. Two capsules per day should be sufficient.

SOME OTHER USES

Among many other uses, the Chinese also use garlic in the treatment of hypertension and heart conditions, but these are dealt with in a later chapter. They also claim that it can be helpful in certain female disorders, particularly menstrual cramps. In *Secrets of the Chinese Herbalists*, a report is given of a lady who had severe menstrual cramps on the first two days of each period. Since she started to take garlic perles she claims that these have been reduced to a minor condition. This particular patient took four or five perles on each day of menstruation and two or three every other day.

It is not only in China and the East that the use of garlic is still popular. In North America and throughout Europe the use of garlic is on the increase and as research continues, more scientific explanations for the old superstitions and benefits in herbal experience are becoming available, convincing many sceptics that this really is a valuable remedy.

Russian scientists treat garlic very seriously indeed and use it as an alternative to penicillin in many cases. In fact, such is the strength of their faith in garlic that it is often referred to as Russian Penicillin. In England too, many herbalists still recommend garlic extensively and this practice is growing as more information becomes available. Its effectiveness across a wide spectrum of conditions can be seen from the following reports which have been received from practising herbalists and proprieters of health food stores. These are not scientific reports but are the honest and sincere opinions of people who have recommended garlic and observed the results, which have given them a conviction in its value.

SOME REPORTED BENEFITS

One of the most respected men in herbal medicine in the United Kingdom today is Professor Shellard who for many years taught herbal medicine to students of pharmacy at Chelsea College, London. In a recent conversation with him he told me a story which he claims he used to relate to his students. He would pose the following hypothetical question: 'What three things would you take with you if you were stranded on a desert island?' His own choice was opium, garlic and rhubarb. I am not sure how serious he was about the opium and rhubarb but he certainly was very convincing when he spoke about garlic. Professor Shellard also told me of his own experience of its anti-bactericidal properties and how its broad area of activity makes it so helpful in the treatment of disease. On one occasion he was visiting Poland when he contracted a bacterial infection affecting his intestines and garlic succeeded in clearing it up when other methods had failed. He also told me that for coughs he always uses a preparation containing garlic.

I am indebted to Mr T. G. Nordal a Member of the National Institute of Herbalists who has a practice in West London, for permission to quote from the following letter:

> The use of garlic is thousands of years old and only recently, in the medical press, there was a doctor writing that he had 'discovered' the excellent properties of garlic!
>
> In my practice garlic oil is used for its many properties, amongst which are its antiseptic qualities, anti-bacteriostatic, expectorant, diuretic, diaphoretic and cleansing properties.
>
> In our family most of us have been or are doctors or vets, and I suppose that I am part of the

first generation of 'medical herbalists'. It is interesting to note that the other doctors in our family are also very herb orientated. Garlic oil is used in my practice as an aid to preventing winter colds and influenza, also lung complaints. From October to March I advocate the taking of garlic oil capsules, as one finds that the patient remains free from colds, or if a cold is caught, only a mild inconvenience usually results. Thus, it is a good winter preventative.

In the treatment of the lungs it has much to offer, especially in cases of haemoptysis and pulmonary tuberculosis. It helps to ease coughs and ease the mucous membrane. It reduces temperatures and is useful in asthma, bronchitis and catarrh.

A very valuable remedy for the treatment of circulatory problems, heart and liver, as well as arteries, capilliaries and veins. Ideal for the digestive processes and for the removal of toxic products of metabolism. Intestinal mucous membrane is toned and peristalsis is aided. It often removes the pain of swollen breasts.

Mr Nordal closes his very comprehensive lists of conditions which respond to garlic with the comment that garlic oil capsules have 1001 uses. His letter is certainly a powerful testament to the very wide range of problems which are safely treated by herbalists with garlic.

It is also interesting to note the claim that it is a first class winter ailment preventative. A great many people take garlic oil capsules regularly throughout the year, but particularly during the winter months when there are so many infections about. In medicine prevention is always better than cure and there are many recorded references to cases where the preventative benefits of taking a course of garlic capsules have helped patients to avoid the common winter ailments.

Miss E. Uttley who runs the health food store in Scarborough tells of a gentleman who had suffered from bronchitis for many years and who, when he was in his sixties, started to take garlic perles regularly. He reports that nothing had helped him so much previously and that a wonderful difference occurred when he started to take garlic regularly.

She also tells of a lady who had regular hospital check-ups for high blood pressure. She commenced taking garlic perles for catarrhal congestion which was greatly relieved. She also noticed that, although she was not taking any other additional medicine to that previously prescribed, her blood pressure fell and stayed down during this period.

From Llanelli in Wales, Mrs F. G. Bennett of Jelf's Health and Herbal Stores writes about two cases. The first, a lady of eighty-two years, kept herself free from bronchitis by taking garlic perles from September to May. The second case was of an overweight husband and wife who were taking garlic for chest complaints and who both lost a stone while taking the treatment. Mrs Bennett reports that in her region of West Wales garlic is taken mainly for catarrh and chest complaints.

In Scotland Mr Anderson of the health food store in Dunfermline states that he has always recommended garlic for bronchial and respiratory troubles. He goes on to explain that as customers return he asks them how they have found the treatment and whether they have obtained any other benefits. The following is a list of complaints which people have told him have been helped by garlic: eczema, blood pressure, arthritis, catarrhal complaints and circulatory problems. All these complaints were either completely cleared up or considerably helped when garlic perles were taken regularly.

Dr Moyhudin who has a successful consultancy practice based on health food stores in Bolton, Bury, Burnley and Oldham in Lancashire, also recommends garlic for colds and sinus congestion. Additionally he prescribes it together with other nutrients for hypertension and, because of its anti-bacterial properties, advocates its use internally for the treatment of acne and boils.

Mr Ernest Winterbottom, the Centre Manager of the Wessex Healthy Living Foundation, Bournemouth, writes that he has known for many years of the use of garlic oil in the treatment of rheumatism and catarrh. He relates a personal family experience that, after many months of failure with pills of all kinds from the doctor, his godson was cleared of worms in ten days. He took garlic capsules, washed down with hot tea before breakfast and the worms were quickly eliminated.

Mr Winterbottom also tells of another quite remarkable case:

> A lady brought to me a very old dog with ear canker. A golden Labrador who had raised many hundreds of pounds for charity, she was in a very distressed state and the left ear was running with black slime. I broke two garlic capsules into a tablespoonful of sunflower seed oil and very gently cleaned out the ear. Afterwards I punctured another capsule and gently dropped the contents, one drop at a time, as far down the ear as I could.
>
> The owner brought the dog back the following week for another treatment. The dog came in by herself and put her head on my knee, with the infected ear uppermost. There was no need for her to return a third time, the condition was completely cleared.

From Northern Ireland, Mr J. Morrison of Belfast also reports the use of garlic for nasal and bronchial catarrh and in the treatment of rheumatism. He also mentions its beneficial effect upon cholesterol and this subject is covered later in the book.

Other reports of the successful use and versatility of garlic can be found in health magazines. Leon Chaitow, a naturopath and osteopath writing about bronchitis in the January 1980 edition of the *Here's Health* magazine says that 'the use of garlic has long been advocated as being of value in both acute and chronic episodes of catarrh.' He goes on to describe garlic's antibiotic properties and how it appears to loosen thick catarrhal obstructions. He recommends garlic in the diet or, as an alternative, four to eight garlic capsules to be taken each day.

Katie Boyle, the well known T.V. and Radio personality, writes regularly for *Here's Health* and in the July 1979 edition, in an article about the subject of leg cramps at night she says, 'Many people swear that keeping corks, magnets and a number of other things between the sheets puts an end to the complaint, but the remedy I've heard the most successful reports of consists of taking garlic perles.'

Betty Lee Morales is one of America's leading writers on natural health problems. She has a regular column in the *Let's Live* magazine and recently in an answer to a letter from a reader who had a problem with tape worms, she related the story about a man who called her to report that he had passed an enormous tapeworm without any stress or illness. This man had taken four capsules of garlic oil after each of three meals daily plus four more at bedtime. He had also had a warm water enema containing a liquid garlic preparation. In the same article Miss Morales tells of the many people who suffer from high blood pressure and who take garlic to control it. She also tells of others who recommend it for circulatory problems.

ARTHRITIS AND RHEUMATISM

In practically all countries where there is a history of herbal medicine, the use of garlic in the treatment of rheumatism and associated diseases is recorded. This is certainly true of Russia were garlic is extensively used in the treatment of such problems. Recent experiments in Japan tested a garlic extract on patients with lumbago and arthritis and a large number of patients benefited without any undesirable side effects. Garlic has been shown to exhibit an anti-inflammatory property which could account for its effectiveness in the treatment of arthritis and rheumatism.

Many herbal practitioners in Britain regularly recommend garlic to rheumatic sufferers. The most popular method is to take the garlic perles internally, although some reports also indicate that pain can be relieved by rubbing the affected parts with cloves of cut garlic. Garlic oil is rapidly absorbed through the skin and into the bloodstream and will quickly reach the affected areas.

The exact method by which garlic is able to relieve rheumatism is still uncertain and there are a number of theories which have been put forward. It is well accepted that garlic is a powerful blood purifier and one school of thought suggests that this is probably the reason why those who take garlic regularly experience relief. Another theory is that rheumatism may be caused by the toxic by-products of virus infection which attack the joints causing rheumatism. Viral infections attack all of us at some time during our life and as children most of us suffer from diseases such as whooping cough, chicken pox or measles and it may be that the results of these childhood infections manifest themselves in later life as rheumatism. Whatever the reason, there is no doubt that a great many people have reported considerable relief from the pain and discomfort caused by rheumatism and similar complaints when they have been taking garlic perles regularly.

DOSAGE

I cannot stress too much the importance of ensuring that the dose of garlic or any other herbal remedy, is taken regularly and for a reasonable period of time. Some people expect herbal medicines to act as quickly and dramatically as powerful drugs. When they have a headache and take an aspirin they expect the pain to be relieved in a matter of minutes and expect herbal medicine to have the same instant effect. Herbs treat the condition not the symptom, they correct the cause, which has possibly taken years to develop and it often needs days or even weeks before any permanent relief is experienced. This is not always the case and garlic, in particular, can and does act quickly especially with colds, catarrh, and intestinal disorders. The important rule to follow is to take the treatment regularly.

DETOXIFYING AGENT

Garlic has also been used successfully for a variety of skin complaints. Dr K. Nolfi explains in her book *My Experiences with Living Food* the results she has achieved. She has established that pimples will disappear without scar when rubbed several times a day with raw garlic. Many other skin disorders including the very persistent form of acne which some adults suffer from, have also been healed with garlic. There have been other instances reported by lay people and medical practitioners, describing how garlic can help to clear the skin of spots and pimples and boils, but in all cases it is clear that, unless the blood is purified then the symptoms will return. Garlic should, therefore, also be taken internally by any person who wants long-term clearance of the skin. Because of its established properties as a powerful detoxifier and cleanser of the blood, garlic is the first herbal treatment to try in most instances of skin problems. A regular course of three garlic perles per day should help to clear minor skin infections quickly. More serious problems may require the advice of a herbal consultant.

The blood purifying and detoxifying effects of garlic on the body, have often been noticed by doctors. Garlic neutralizes toxins, not just in the blood but also in the digestive tract and the beneficial action on other organs, especially the liver, kidneys, nervous system and circulation have naturally brought about general improvements in the health of patients.

A Japanese study clearly demonstrates the protective and detoxifying effect of garlic. In these trials a group of rats were fed on a diet, to which was added five per cent sodium cyclamate, an artificial sweetener. This diet had an adverse effect on the rats who exhibited a slowing down of growth and weight gain, poor hair condition and extensive diarrhoea. A second group of rats were given the same diet to which had been added a special garlic extract. These rats grew healthy and strong and to almost twice the size of the rats which did not receive garlic. This demonstrated that garlic, through its detoxifying properties, had been able to protect the second group of rats from the toxic effects of the cyclamate.

Food additives, artificial colourings, sweeteners and many other chemicals are present in the food we eat; chemical pesticides and fertilizers which are used on the farm sometimes remain as traces in the food and so are still present when we consume it. The result is that all these chemicals accumulate in the body, upsetting the natural balance and possibly giving rise to illness. Garlic can help to neutralize these toxic products and protect our body from the harmful effects.

ALLERGIES

There is an increasing amount of evidence that the chemicals used in just about everything we come into contact with in daily life can affect our health. It is not just what we eat, but also what we breath and touch which can upset the body. Allergies can result from a whole host of chemicals, most particularly those which are derived from petroleum. This gives rise to many allergy symptoms which can be most distressing and the cause is often difficult to trace.

Not all allergies fall into this class and many such as hay fever are due to natural causes. Garlic has been found helpful to many people who suffer from allergies. Bert Lenthall, the sales manager of Lusty's Natural Products Limited, one of the leading companies supplying garlic perles, told me of a lady who had approached him at an exhibition in Plymouth to express her appreciation for the help that Lusty's Garlic Perles had been to her daughter. This lady volunteered the information that her daughter had suffered for many months from an allergy with symptoms similar to hay fever, i.e. watering eyes, running nose, sneezing, etc. She had been taking antihistamine drugs from her doctor in an attempt to control the allergy. These drugs, however, made her daughter drowsy and had, in fact, spoiled their annual summer holiday because the girl felt so lethargic. She was recommended by a herbal consultant to take garlic perles and a dose of three per day quickly helped to clear the unpleasant symptoms, without any undesirable side effects.

This lady also claimed that when the perles were taken with hot water, her daughter experienced no after taste and her breath did not smell of garlic. Others have reported the same effect if they are taken with lemon juice. For most people however this is not a problem, the modern method of taking garlic in the form of soft gelatine capsules gives rise to very few cases where garlic gives offence.

Allergies are peculiar conditions to deal with because the cause is often very difficult to isolate. Similar sets of symptoms can be due to totally different circumstances. Garlic is not a certain cure for all the many different allergies that exist, but it is certainly worth a try and can do no harm.

AS A PREVENTATIVE

The above examples of the very many ways in which garlic has and is still being used in the treatment of diseases of all types, illustrates what a versatile medicinal herb it is. Effective as it is in so many diverse ways, its greatest value is still perhaps its ability to help *prevent* disease. Preventative medicine depends for its success on regular usage and if this is done then garlic will reward by helping to prevent many illnesses. People who take garlic regularly have often commented that even when they have been exposed to infection or virus's, then their body has been able to throw off the illness quickly and without difficulty. A regular dose of one garlic perle three times per day can do much to help prevent illness, keeping the body fit and healthy.

GARLIC AND THE HEALTH OF YOUR PETS

Just as garlic can help prevent disease in man and is an effective cure from a wide range of complaints, so it can also help animals to stay fit and healthy. In the wild, sick animals have to be their own doctors. If they are injured or diseased they will often seek out wild herbs and eat them, even carnivorous animals will often supplement their diet with plants and grasses. Domestic pets are not free to find natural cures for themselves, but their owners can do much to ensure that they too receive the benefits of natural herbal medicines.

One of the leading authorities on herbal medicines and natural diets for domestic pets is Buster Lloyd-Jones. He has written a number of books on natural animal care and is a great advocate of garlic, particularly for worming. In a recent article Mr Lloyd-Jones described his experiences of thirty years use of garlic for treating worms in dogs and cats. There is a tiny parasitic worm carried by dogs and this not only causes distress to the animal but it can also be passed to humans through the animal's excrement. Some methods of dealing with worms are very harsh and can lead to gastro-enteritis and weakened bowels in the animal. Garlic, being a natural herbal medicine is gentle and safe and will act as an internal disinfectant, quickly removing worms and leaving the dog or cat healthy and happy.

One company, Denes of Hove, Sussex specialize in the supply of natural medicines for animals and these are available from Health Food Stores. They produce an excellent booklet called *Natural Health For Your Pets* which is written by Buster Lloyd-Jones and gives a lot of first-class advice to pet owners on how their pets can be reared on a natural diet and how their ailments can be treated with the use of herbal medicines. It recommends that garlic be used externally for abscesses and to clean cuts and bites and internally for inflammed glands, lack of appetite, asthma, ear canker, to keep coat in good condition diarrhoea, fleas, gastritis and rheumatism. However, there is no doubt that above all else its use as a treatment for worms it is without equal in the field of natural cures. Denes also recommend garlic as a preventative medicine to help build up the animal's resistance to disease and particularly to help prevent worms and clear catarrhal conditions.

If you require further information about the use of garlic and other natural medicines and diets for use with domestic animals, you may write to Denes Veterinary Products Limited, 14 Goldstone Street, Hove, East Sussex.

The garlic used for pets is the same as for humans and if you are already using garlic then one or two perles will usually be enough as a dose for pets. If your pet will not swallow capsules then they can be pierced with a pin and the contents squeezed into water or onto food.

SUMMARY

H. A. Hoppe in a well respected and authoritative German herbal textbook, *Drogen Kunde*, lists the following uses made of garlic in medicine. I can find no other better way to summarize the versatility of this wonderful herb than by including it at the end of this chapter.

1. Prevents arteriosclerosis and hypertension (high blood pressure).
2. Because of its antibacterial activity is used to treat illness of the stomach and intestines.
3. Active against streptococci, staphylococci and bacteria causing certain kinds of typhoid and dysentery.
4. Promotes bile secretions.
5. Protects against stomach upsets, especially when travelling abroad, when changes of climate, water and diet can be disturbing.
6. Preventative medicine against flu virus, colds, etc.
7. Used against nicotine poisoning.
8. Treats various skin disorders.
9. Eliminates worm infections.
10. Anti-fungal properties make it a good treatment for athletes foot.
11. Allicin is active against both gram-negative and gram-positive micro-organisms.
12. Juice used to treat wounds.
13. Appetite stimulant.

CHAPTER FIVE

THE CLINICAL EVIDENCE

Having considered the many ways in which garlic has been used in the kitchen and particularly as a medicine, it is now time to examine its chemical structure and to try and discover how, and why it is so effective in the treatment and prevention of disease. Herbalists have known for centuries that garlic cured illness, but I think it fair to state that it is only since the First World War that extensive scientific research has been undertaken to investigate the properties which make garlic such an effective medicine. This interest probably sprang from the very successful use of garlic in cases of gangrene and other extremely serious wound infections during the 1914–18 war. It is claimed that garlic was primarily responsible for lowering the incidence of sceptic poisoning among wounded soldiers in the Second World War. The undoubted antiseptic properties, like its other remedial properties, have now been scientifically investigated.

ACTIVE FACTORS IN GARLIC
Garlic is an extremely complex herb containing a vast number of chemical compounds, but by far the most important of these from the medical point of view are those which contain sulphur. There are thirty-three such sulphur compounds which have so far been isolated from the simple garlic corm, of these the most significant are allicin, alliin and the enzyme allinase. Dr Paavo Airola in his book *The*

Miracle of Garlic lists ten active 'factors' which are present in garlic and responsible for some or all of its many activities. These are:

Allicin
This substance is believed to be largely responsible for giving garlic its anti-bacterial and anti-inflammatory effect.

Alliin
Garlic is often known as Russian Penicillin and the Russians believe, as do many other scientists, that this is the substance which produces its antibiotic activity.

Di-sulphides
These are believed to have a cholesterol lowering effect which help garlic to control cholesterol and other fats within the arteries and blood vessels.

Anti-haemolytic Factor
It is claimed that this is responsible for the beneficial effect of garlic in the treatment of anaemia.

Anti-arthritic Factor
Japanese research teams investigating arthritis and similar conditions, claim this factor to be present in garlic.

Sugar Regulating Factor
It was reported in the *Lancet* in 1973 that garlic was useful for treating some forms of diabetes. It is claimed this factor is responsible.

Anti-oxidant Factor
Garlic has been shown capable of helping to prevent foods from going rancid.

Anti-coagulant Factor
Garlic contains certain active substances which appear to prevent blood from coagulating therefore benefiting certain heart conditions.

Allithiamin
This special type of vitamin B_1 has been isolated from garlic and has beneficial properties.

Selenium

This is a trace element very similar in its anti-oxidant action to vitamin E and therefore useful in heart conditions. Other research workers have attributed additional active factors to garlic. It contains a substance called scordinine, which is very similar to the male and female hormones and is also found in ginseng herbs. It may be responsible for a number of activities in the body, particularly what is referred to as 'normalization' of body functions. This means that it can lower the blood pressure in high blood pressure sufferers and increase it in cases of low blood pressure. In other words it can return it to normal. The same appears to be true of different body functions, not just blood pressure.

As with all natural products the content of these factors in garlic will vary depending on the origin, type of soil in which it is grown, climate, time of harvesting and how it has been stored and treated since harvesting. The method of extraction of the oil can also determine the content of its health-giving properties. This refers to raw garlic and one advantage of the garlic perles is that the oil content can be checked and standardized so that it consistently contains a proper balance.

ALLIIN, ALLINASE AND ALLICIN

When garlic is freshly harvested it is virtually odourless and, as I have said, the characteristic pungent odour is the result of the action of an enzyme. An enzyme is a substance which produces a chemical reaction in a cell without itself being changed. The substance in garlic called alliin is converted by the action of an enzyme, allinase into allicin. Both alliin and allinase are present in the cells of the garlic corm, but they are in separate 'compartments' and it is only when the corm is cut or bruised that the two come into contact. When this happens a spontaneous chemical reaction takes place and the alliin is converted, by the allinase, into allicin. It is in the form of allicin that one of the most powerful active principles of garlic works within the body's system and it is allicin that has the anti-bacterial activity which is attributed to garlic. Cooking destroys allinase and this is why cooked garlic has a less strong odour, providing it is cooked whole.

Although garlic is one of the oldest medicines known to man, it was only in the 1940s that the active substance alliin was isolated by chemical experiment. Dr Stoll, a Nobel Prizewinner from Switzerland was the scientist responsible for the discovery. Further research produced evidence of the enzymatic action which is necessary for the conversion of alliin to allicin. Allicin, which is responsible for the anti-bactericidal action of garlic, is so powerful that it is active in concentrations as low as one part per hundred thousand, still strong enough at this dilution to destroy many micro-organisms, especially gram-negative types which are responsible for the bacterial infections which are most difficult to treat. Garlic has the further advantage of being a natural remedy which is effective even against some forms of bacteria that ordinary antibiotics will not treat. One of the problems with conventional antibiotics is that they can cause the body to build up antibodies which counteract the effect of the drug, and prolonged use of them can make them ineffective, the body builds up a resistance to them. This does not happen with garlic and many people believe that it would be far better to treat minor infections with garlic rather than a more powerful antibiotic, and so save the power of the conventional drugs to tackle really serious problems.

SULPHUR

Both alliin and allicin are sulphur containing chemical compounds and garlic contains many other sulphur based compounds. Sulphur itself is an extremely important mineral although it is not particularly well understood despite the fact that it is one of the very oldest chemical elements used as a remedy. Within the human body sulphur is found in the muscles, joints, bone, cartilage, and significant amounts are present in the hair, skin and nails. Nutritional deficiencies of sulphur give rise to a number of disorders e.g. many skin problems can be traced to a lack of sulphur, these include psoriasis, rashes, eczema and spots. The condition of the hair may also indicate a sulphur deficiency, for example, when the hair is greying, going thin or growing slowly. Because sulphur is a necessary nutrient for the joints and muscles it has often been linked with the theory that rheumatism and arthritis can be due to deficiency diseases, if this were found to be correct, then without doubt, a sulphur deficiency could be the cause of some forms of rheumatism and arthritis.

Sulphur also acts as a detoxifier of the blood and a general body 'cleanser', helping to remove toxins and other waste products from the body. It can also act as a laxative and has been reported to be capable of checking the growth of some types of parasites.

Many of these conditions are of course similar to those which we have already seen can be treated successfully with garlic. Undoubtedly the high sulphur content in garlic helps to make it such a powerful medicine. However, it is not merely the presence of sulphur, but rather the very special and complex forms in which it exists in garlic that distinguish it from elemental sulphur or other sulphur containing compounds.

Most scientists today, seem to agree that it is these di-sulphides, particularly allicin, which have the properties which make garlic an effective medicine. Various theories are put forward to try and explain the exact method by which these compounds act and arguments for and against are extremely technical ones. Research continues to try and discover as much as possible about the ingredients that are present in garlic and, as well as this, there is a great deal of medical research being undertaken, with clinical trials and long-term experiments, designed to try to assess and prove garlic's potential in treating the 'diseases of civilization'. These are the diseases that rich western nations suffer from and which are unknown to primitive tribes. Many of them are illnesses which were unknown in Britain and America at the beginning of the century but which now kill or cripple millions every year. In particular, heart diseases and hypertension have increased dramatically over the past eighty years and have reached the level when heart disease is now the number one killer in many countries.

GARLIC AGAINST HEART DISEASE

There is now accumulating a growing body of evidence to support the contention that garlic, through one of its many forms of action within the body, can help to control the incidence of heart disease. Once again it illustrates how the ancient healers found a cure which, until now, we were unable to prove. Dioscorides, the ancient Greek physician wrote thousands of years ago that 'garlic doth clear the arteries'. The ancient healers did not possess one single fact about the chemistry of garlic but obviously they had somehow stumbled across its ability to help the health of the arteries. Throughout the 1970s there has been a number of medical papers published in journals throughout the world which support the claim that garlic can and does influence the arteries, the blood cholesterol level and high blood pressure, which are all linked to heart disease.

Cholesterol Levels

When the arteries of heart attack patients are examined in the post-mortems a great number contain fatty deposits which have built up on the artery walls. It is a well accepted fact that these deposits of cholesterol and other fats are one of the prime causative factors leading to heart attacks. They cause arteriosclerosis and the statistics show that when this condition exists, the patient is more prone to heart attack and high blood pressure. One of the principal fats involved is cholesterol, but there are other fats (or lipids) which also contribute to the narrowing of the arteries. These deposits restrict the flow of blood to the heart and brain and make clots of blood more likely to block the flow, causing a stroke or heart attack. As we shall see the progress that has been made during the 1970s shows that there is a good possibility that garlic will help to protect from these killer diseases.

Not only does garlic seem able to help combat the build-up of fatty deposits in the arteries but it also helps to make the blood less 'sticky'. Modern clinical investigation has indicated that garlic can help prevent fats, which circulate in the bloodstream, from sticking together. When these tiny droplets or 'platelets' of blood agglomerate, they form lumps or clots which in turn block up the arteries. If a fatty deposit is present on the walls of the blood vessels, then these blockages occur much more easily. Garlic seems to make these platelets less sticky.

Two doctors, Bordia and Bansal, wrote to the well respected medical journal *Lancet* in 1973 to publish the results of trials which they had undertaken using garlic in an attempt to prove whether or not it could be helpful in treating heart disease. Their report concluded that garlic could be recommended for long-term use, without any danger of toxicity, and that it did in fact lower blood cholesterol levels.

In *Herbs that Heal*, (Black, London) Dr William Thomson tells how a whole series of tests into garlic's potential in heart conditions probably started with a chance remark. Apparently, a patient mentioned that in France when horses develop clots in the legs they are often given a diet containing garlic and onion. The doctors picked up this casual remark and set in motion a chain of research that still continues and which is helping to give a scientific understanding for what, at first reading, appears to be just another folk tale.

There are many potent modern drugs which are used to treat heart conditions but none of them can claim to be free from side-effects. Garlic as a preventative therapy has no ill effects and can do nothing but good.

Drs Bordia and Bansal selected ten healthy patients and tested their average blood cholesterol. Before the trials commenced this averaged 221. The ten were fed a very fatty diet which included a high proportion of animal fats known to be rich in cholesterol, after three hours the blood cholesterol level had reached 237. Cholesterol levels were allowed to return to normal and the subjects were then given the same high fat diet, but this time they also included garlic or garlic oil. Instead of the blood cholesterol levels increasing by an average of 16, they dropped by 16 points. This seems to provide proof that garlic is not only able to control an increase but, even more significant, is capable of bringing about a reduction in the amount of cholesterol circulating in the blood.

Blood Clotting

Dr Bordia was also interested in what happened to the blood clotting time, that is the period taken for blood to start to form into lumps or clots. It is essential that blood starts to clot when we cut ourself, in order to arrest the bleeding, but when clotting occurs in the arteries it can cause angina, heart attacks or strokes. There is a substance in the blood called fibrin which in effect ties up the sticky globules of blood into clots. Garlic can protect against spontaneous clotting by making the platelets of blood less sticky, so that they do not form clots so easily and it also promotes the natural blood processes which help to dissolve clots once they have started to form.

Dr Bordia took blood samples from six volunteers and tested the time it took for the blood to start clotting. He then repeated the process, adding garlic oil to the samples and again tested the difference in time taken for the blood to clot. Garlic was able to help prevent the platelets from sticking together and when it was added *after* the blood had started to form into lumps, it started to dissolve them.

The doctor then decided to test the results of

his experiments, which up to this point had been done in test tubes, within the human body. Volunteers were given a diet which included approximately 25 mg of garlic oil every day. He tested the time it took for the platelets to come together, then five days later repeated the tests. In all cases there was an increase in the time taken for the platelets to start to form into clots; convincing proof that garlic really can influence the action of the blood.

Another doctor who has done a lot of work with garlic and published many papers about its cholesterol lowering abilities, is Dr Jain. Dr Jain's first experiments involved feeding a high cholesterol diet to rabbits. He was able to show that those who had received a high cholesterol diet without garlic had suffered nearly double the build up of cholesterol deposits in the arteries leading to the heart, compared to those which had received the same diet but with the addition of garlic.

Dr Jain later carried out further experiments in an attempt to repeat the results in human beings. He was able to feed a group of subjects with a diet that included garlic every day. The tests were carried out over three weeks and at the end of each week Dr Jain examined the levels of various fats in the blood. He found that there had been a gradual lowering of blood cholesterol levels over this short period of time.

RECENT RESEARCH

Modern studies have indicated that there are two types of cholesterol circulating in the blood i.e. a high density and low density cholesterol. It is now believed that it is the low density cholesterol which carries most risk of heart disease. Dr Jain's experiments showed that the type of cholesterol which garlic reduced was, in tact, this low density cholesterol. At the English College, Valladolid, Spain, Dr David L. Greenstock, the Director of the Biological Research Laboratory stated that the experiments they have conducted into the anit-coagulant and cholesterol lowering properties of garlic have confirmed the findings of Dr Jain. Dr Greenstock, says: 'Investigations into the anti-coagulant properties brought good results with no room for reasonable doubt. We have proved its effect on serum lipids, reduction of the cholesterol index and coagulability.'

Another letter to *Lancet* in 1976 reported on an investigation conducted with three separate groups of patients, who ate different diets. Apart from diet, the groups were as closely matched as possible. Group 1 were given a mixed diet which contained quite large amounts of garlic and onion. Group 2 were strict vegetarians who had never eaten garlic and group 3 were also strict vegetarians but did eat small amounts of garlic and onion regularly. Various tests were conducted on blood samples taken from each group and the results analysed. The researchers concluded that the regular consumption of garlic and onion in the diet seemed to have a protective effect against some of the factors which influence atherosclerosis, such as blood fats and blood coagulation times.

In 1978 *Doctor* published an article which reported the comments of Professor Hans Reuter of Cologne, West Germany. The professor stated that there is proof that garlic, taken regularly, can help clear cholesterol from the blood of those whose diet is rich in fatty foods. Tests showed that garlic oil capsules controlled the blood cholesterol levels in volunteers. Professor Reuter is also reported to believe that as well as driving out fats in the blood, garlic acts as an antibiotic which, in certain circumstances, can be more effective than penicillin.

GARLIC AND HIGH BLOOD PRESSURE

Garlic also figures in recent experiments designed to show that it could help to reduce high blood pressure. Dr Paavo Airola in *The Miracle of Garlic* claims that, in his own medical practice, patients with high blood pressure had reacted well to large doses of garlic preparations and in most cases blood pressure was reduced by 20–30 mm in one week. Experiments in animals have shown that garlic could reduce blood pressure and one of the first researchers to confirm that the same was true in humans, was Dr F. G. Piotrowski. Working at the University of Geneva, he used garlic on 100 patients suffering from abnormally high blood pressure. In 40 per cent of the cases treated there was a significant reduction in blood pressure within one week of the treatment commencing. Dr Piotrowski claimed that garlic had a dilatory effect on the blood vessels, that is, it had the effect of making them wider, thus reducing the pressure. If this action does in fact occur, then it would partially explain why garlic is so helpful in the treatment of arteriosclerosis, for the dilatory effect would allow the blood to flow more freely.

The Chinese herbalists have used garlic for many years to normalize both high and low blood pressure. They believe that the type of blood pressure characterized by symptoms of dizziness, lack of concentration, ringing in the ears and hypertension caused by arteriosclerosis, responds well to treatment with garlic. Other forms of blood pressure, such as that caused by kidney disease, do not seem to respond and in these cases garlic is of little value. Richard Lucas, in *Secrets of the Chinese Herbalists*, writes that the herbalists use either fresh garlic or garlic oil in the form of perles or capsules to relieve high blood pressure. The dosage is usually from one to three perles, swallowed with water three times daily. Once the blood pressure has been brought under control and reduced to an acceptable level the dosage can be reduced to maintain the improvement.

Dr Nolfi in her book *My Experiences with Living Food* reports that garlic lowers high blood pressure, raises blood pressure which is too low, but leaves normal pressure unaffected. Other reports of the successful use of the herb come from doctors in France, Germany and throughout Europe, all testifying to the remarkable power of garlic and its ability to correct high blood pressure and to treat heart diseases.

GARLIC AS AN ANTIBIOTIC

The August 1979 edition of *Prevention* magazine published by Rodale Press, gives reports from two countries where there has been an attempt to prove experimentally, the extent of the antibiotic properties of garlic. It is not easy to obtain up-to-date scientific information from Russia, but there is a report in a Russian journal concerning an extract of garlic called phytocidin. The extract was applied to various types of bacteria including those which are responsible for tuberculosis and diphtheria. Garlic was shown to have an antibiotic effect on all the different types of bacteria which were tested.

From Greece another study indicates that a 5 per cent concentration of garlic was effective against *Staphylococcus aureus*, a very vigorous and persistent strain of bacteria which is often responsible for food poisoning.

One research establishment which has done a tremendous amount of work on the antibiotic properties of various garlic extracts is the Biological Research Laboratory at the English College in Spain. The director of the laboratory, Dr Greenstock has made a long and detailed study of garlic and is himself in the course of preparing a book describing the work that has been undertaken in his laboratories. I am extremely grateful to Dr Greenstock for making available some of the results of his work in the field and for his kind permission to include a summary of the laboratory's findings in this book.

One of the things they set out to determine was the extent of the antibiotic properties of various garlic extracts against toxic producing bacteria. This they have successfully achieved and, in addition, they also found that garlic did no harm to friendly bacteria which exist in the intestines and which have a beneficial, even essential, function. What is more they have not come across any harmful side effects, even after long periods of garlic administration. In all the time they have been researching garlic they have only noticed one case of allergy which could be shown to be caused by garlic extracts. Dr Greenstock reports that they have tested garlic extracts against fifteen different types of toxic bacteria, including the very resistant strain of *Staphylococcus aureus*, and in all cases garlic was found to be an effective antibiotic.

One of the most encouraging aspects of these results is the absence of known side-effects. Compare this to the many well known side effects of conventional antibiotic drugs. Even after long periods of using therapeutic quantities of garlic and with a very thorough follow-up programme over five to ten years, no side-effects have been noticed. However, in the case of one type of disease, which affects the gums around the roots of the teeth (a disease incidentally which has responded well to garlic therapy) and where treatment has to cover a long period of time, some patients do experience a dryness of the mouth.

Dr Greenstock emphasizes that the important element in the garlic therapy is that it is so highly selective against those bacteria which produce toxins, whilst leaving the beneficial intestinal flora intact.

Researchers at Valladolid noticed one very interesting and important fact when carrying out their experiments and that is that garlic seems to have a beneficial effect on the whole organism. As they say, 'its general effect is far beyond any substance known to us at the present moment.' They found that those who undertake garlic therapy, for various reasons, do not develop colds, influenza or intestinal infections. It has also given excellent results against chronic bronchitis and they say that it is probably the best vaccine available at the moment as a preventative against the common cold.

These comments form one of the most powerful and persuasive arguments for taking garlic as a preventative medicine that I have come across. Dr Greenstock and his team continue with their work in Spain and I am sure that my readers will join with me in wishing them success.

Many other experimenters have shown how garlic is able to destroy various types of bacteria. In addition to its previously mentioned action against staphylococci, tests have shown that it is able to destroy both gram-negative and gram-positive micro-organisms including strepto-cocci and bacteria which are responsible for dysentery, enteritis, cholera and typhoid. Russian experiments have introduced garlic extracts into cultures of bacteria and within three minutes the bacteria ceased to function. In 1969 Johnson and Vaughan found garlic to be an effective anti-bacterial agent against salmonella which cause food poisoning and diarrhoea and Ecolli which causes urine infections. It is said that the late Dr Schweitzer used garlic to cure cholera and typhus and, with modern knowledge, it is now easy to understand how and why garlic was so effective in the terrible plagues of long ago.

SUMMARY

These very brief reviews are just a small number of the many experiments which have taken place all over the world in the past few years and which have proved, very convincingly, that garlic meets the need for a powerful, natural, healing medicine which is free from side-effects. In the *Pharmaceutical Journal* of June 1979 a review of papers indicating a new interest in the therapeutic compounds in garlic, covered almost 30 scientific papers of interest to pharmacisists, which gave details of serious scientific experiments that are doing a great deal to confirm the beliefs that have been held for centuries.

Garlic, having fallen from favour a hundred years ago is once more being taken seriously by the medical profession.

There are powerful, modern synthetic drugs and medicaments which can do all the things that garlic is capable of doing. It would be wrong to suppose or suggest that there is no place in medicine for many of these drugs; undoubtedly there is. But the fact remains that, in many cases, treatment with the humble garlic herb could be used in place of antibiotics and other drugs. The use of a natural plant medicine would eliminate the risks of unpleasant side-effects and the build up of resistance to anti-biotics that occurs. In this way the powerful drugs can be saved for the real emergencies when swift and potent action is vital. Current interest in the use of plant based medicine is so strong that we are certain to learn a lot more in the coming years about garlic's ability to cure disease. What is almost equally certain is that we are unlikely to hear of any new use for garlic, which has not already been tried by the healers and herbalists of old for, as we have seen, during its 4,000-year history garlic has been used to treat almost every adverse condition known to man. What we shall discover is an explanation for the beliefs that have been held for so long. Science will eventually teach us how and why garlic is so effective but, in the meantime this 'old fashioned' remedy will carry on as always, treating and curing, healing and preventing so many diseases, just as it has done since the Babylonians first started to use it all those centuries ago.

CHAPTER SIX

HERBAL MEDICINE TODAY

It comes as a great surprise to many people to learn that garlic and many other herbs are still in regular use today. Herbal medicine is often thought of as an out-of-date method of dealing with illness and disease. There is, however, a growing number of people who are returning to natural methods of health care and this often means the use of vitamins, health foods and herbs. Even conventional medical thinking recognizes the need for self-medication and the treatment of the less serious complaints by the individual in his own home. With the growing concern about many of the powerful drugs used today, the return to more natural forms of self-healing has accelerated. Aspirin, paracetamol, phenacetin were until recently available in any retail outlet in large numbers. Today, however, their sale is restricted and they are only available outside a pharmacy in small quantities, in order to prevent misuse.

MEDICAL ATTITUDES
There are many schools of thought about the various types of medicament which ought to be used and many 'fringe' medical systems have been developed. There are opposing views about herbal medicine. On the one hand there are those who claim that herbal medicine is the only real method of obtaining truly natural health. At the other extreme, there are those that think that all herbal medicine is quackery and that the only effective and safe drugs are those produced by the pharmaceutical industry.

The truth lies between the two extremes. It is an undoubted fact that many herbs such as garlic have very effective medicinal properties and also that plants have been used as the source of many drugs. Indeed, even today, many of the drugs which are produced by pharmaceutical companies are derived from plants.

Those who criticize the powerful and potent drugs which have been developed in recent years often choose the tragic story of thalidomide to illustrate the harm that drugs can sometimes cause. However it would be incorrect, indeed foolish, to ignore the fact that many drugs are truly lifesavers and that they have an extremely important role to play in health care. The answer for minor ailments must lie with the individual who has the freedom of choice about which drugs to use for self-medication. In more serious illness and disease however, it is sometimes necessary to use the powerful drugs and the skills of the doctor and pharmacist.

THE HERBAL TRADITION

The origins of herbal medicine are lost in the mists of antiquity. Primitive man would have learned to recognize that certain fruits could correct diarrhoea, various leaves or barks could soothe a pain or relieve a cough and, as we have seen from earlier chapters, he very quickly learned that garlic could be beneficial in a great many instances.

Over the centuries a vast store of herbal knowledge was assembled and passed down from generation to generation. We have seen how the early medical practitioners were often priests or priest/physicians. The early practitioners wrote down their knowledge so that it could be transmitted to others and this practice continued with the publishing of herbals in the sixteenth, seventeenth and eighteenth centuries. It may come as a surprise to learn that the practice of producing herbals continues into the 1980s. The British Herbal Medicine Association has recently published the first two parts of a new work, *The British Herbal Pharmacopoeia*. This contains descriptions of very many herbs, prepared by some of the most senior practitioners in the country, who are members of the National Institute of Medical Herbalists. They include professors and pharmacognocists, and much of the information it contains is gathered from the observations of members of the Institute. The committee which prepares the Pharmacopoeia contains botanists, pharmacists, scientists, herbalists and has medical practitioners to advise it. This reference book is now used as a standard text book by many and is relied upon by the Department of Health and Social Security when they review the safety and effectiveness of medicines.

THE HERBAL APPROACH

The medical herbalist is a general practitioner, he is often unhappy about the degree of specialization which exists in much of medicine today. His methods of diagnosis will be similar to those used by a conventional medical practitioner but his method of treatment is, of course, rather different. The herbalist would claim to treat the cause rather than the symptoms. Rather than prescribe the standard drugs and medicines which are available 'off the shelf', he would prefer to prepare a formulation which is specially geared for the individual needs of the patient. He may use the whole plant in his treatment, or just a part of it, such as the leaves, root or bark. It may be dried and powdered; it will often be in the form of a liquid extract prepared from the herb and standardized so that the dosage and proportions of the active constituents are consistent.

Although the practice of herbal medicine is ancient, the herbalists of today make full use of scientific techniques. Herbs are examined under powerful microscopes and very sophisticated analytical equipment is used to identify the herb and the strength of its constituents. In this way it is possible for the skilled expert to be more precise than ever before about the potency, purity and safety of the herbs used today.

Many herbs are dried and sold singly, they can often be purchased in small quantities from health food or herbal shops. The dried herbs are also sold to the professional herbalists who make up their own remedies for each individual patient. One of the leading suppliers of herbal remedies, Potters of Wigan, list over two hundred different kinds of single herbs. An increasingly popular method of obtaining the benefits of herbs is drinking herbal teas. Infusions of herbs have been served for their medicinal properties for many generations, but in recent years the practice has fallen into decline and the common black teas from India, Ceylon and China are the most popular beverages of today. Health food stores now supply many herb teas and these are usually available as single herbs such as peppermint and camomile, but one interesting new range has just been introduced by Symingtons of Edinburgh, the firm who have produced dandelion coffee (another herbal beverage) for over a hundred years. These new teas are combinations of tried and trusted herbs, blended so that they have a medicinal value and purpose. Thus, one tea blend is designed to help you relax and sleep at night, and another to settle the stomach after a meal. Herbal teas are as easy to prepare as ordinary tea and are an efficient method of obtaining the health benefits of herbs.

TABLETS AND CAPSULES

Tablets and capsules are another popular way of administering herbs, one advantage being that they enable concentrated extracts to be combined in precise dosages which can be dispensed on a daily basis without the need for weighing or measuring.

Herbs are also used externally. Comfrey has been used for generations to heal sprains, bruises, swelling and abrasions; rosemary has been used for the care of the hair; witch hazel, to ease irritation and heal cuts and bruises; pilewort, to treat and soothe haemorrhoids; and, as we have discovered in this book, no medicine has a wider application than garlic, both internally and externally.

COSMETICS

Herbs were the very first cosmetic ingredients and are still used today. Shampoos, facial creams and lotions, skin tonics and moisturizers can all be produced from herbal ingredients. Indeed, herbal ingredients have become so popular that many leading cosmetic houses have adopted the use of herbs within the range of products they offer. However, these will almost certainly prove to be fads or fashions and unfortunately very few of them are true herbal concoctions. Although they do contain some herbal matter (otherwise they would contravene the Trades Descriptions Act), the amount present is very often insufficient to have any beneficial effects. There are, however, ranges of cosmetic products available from health food stores which use the time-proven benefits of various herbs such as willow, nettle, thyme, valerian, elder blossom, calendula and witch hazel. One such range, sold under the brand name 'Tiki', contains generous amounts of herbal extracts, sufficient for them to be effective, and is popular among young and old alike. These are certainly not 'fashion conscious' cosmetics, but a serious attempt to use the value of herbs to care for the skin and hair.

HOLISTIC HEALING POWER
The herbal tradition contends that the whole plant has different and more balanced properties than extracts. Some of the criticism that has been levelled at the use of herbal medicine has been a criticism, not of the whole herb but of an extract which has been isolated from the herb and which scientists have believed to be responsible for its curative properties.

An example of this unfair assumption can be found in the herb rauwolfia. This is a root which has been sold in the bazaars of India for centuries for use as a nerve soother. About twenty-five years ago researchers in the West discovered in the herb an active principle which they were able to isolate, that is to say, they removed everything else from the herb except this active ingredient. The resultant drug was used as a treatment for high blood pressure. While it was effective it became apparent that it also had quite severe side-effects which caused depression in some patients and it could be potentially dangerous in others with a weak heart. Rauwolfia itself does not seem to produce these undesirable side-effects, it is only the active principle which pharmacists had isolated from the herb that produced the damaging results.

Often the total effect of the ingredients in a whole herb is quite different from that of an isolated part of the herb administered separately. The whole herb, in the form given to us by nature, is the way that herbs are used by most herbal practitioners.

The same is true of many other herbs. Indeed, as we have seen, garlic contains many active principles and its properties cannot be explained by any one of them in isolation. It is the combined effect of all the component parts which gives the desired effect. This synergistic action explains why the whole herb works, but the part which appears to have the desired effect is either completely ineffective when separated from the whole herb, or conversely, becomes so potent that it assumes toxic properties.

THE SAFETY OF HERBS

One of the criticisms that is levelled at the herbal medicine industry and profession is that many of the plants have not been subject to controlled clinical tests. Some herbs are dangerous and poisonous. These are so hazardous that they must only be used by skilled practitioners and, even then, only with caution. But all the herbs that are offered for general sale through health food stores and other shops can be used with confidence. They have been shown to be safe from established use by thousands of practitioners and their patients over many centuries. These reports are confirmed by modern knowledge and experience and great care and attention is paid to ensure that no harmful effects result from the use of these products.

Drugs are concentrated, potent substances, but herbs are not. Their action is much more gentle, they work far more slowly and often treatment needs to be continued for several weeks and perhaps longer. Very few work in a matter of hours (although garlic can be effective very quickly in some areas of treatment). Often disease is the results of years of gradual deterioration of health and it is not reasonable to suppose that any treatment can remedy such effects instantly. Certainly herbal medicine will not do so. It is not magic, it is a system which will help the body heal itself, but this will very often take time.

The important thing is that the herb is effective and safe. Although it is interesting to discover how it works, this knowledge is not essential, it is the fact that it does, coupled with confidence in its ability and safety which matter.

LEGAL CONTROLS

The practice of herbal medicine has been permitted by law for over 400 years and this protection still exists today. The freedom to practice herbal medicine seemed to be threatened when the Medicines Act 1968 was first proposed. However, thanks to pressure from manufacturers, herbal practitioners, retailers of herbal products and, of course, those who relied on the products they offered, very important provisions were written in to the Medicines Act which allow the practice of herbal medicine to flourish. Herbal medicines will continue to be made available, under the safeguards contained in the Act, and although there will inevitably be changes, the existence of herbs and herbalists is likely to continue.

The Medicines Act itself has brought with it new standards which apply to all producers of medicine, whether they be herbalists or pharmaceutical companies. There has been a new drive to establish even higher standards of manufacture, quality and purity than existed in the past and new knowledge is coming to light which will benefit the user of herbal remedies. We have already seen how modern experiments with garlic are proving some of the old beliefs and how we have learned much more about its component parts. This is typical of the developments which are taking place in the fields of herbal medicine.

POPULARITY AND POTENTIAL

Since plants have been used so successfully as medicines for many centuries, it is not surprising that some of them are still in common use today. It is surprising to learn, however, just how many of the drugs currently prescribed are derived from plants. It is not just the herbalists who use these plant-based drugs but doctors in all fields of medicine. In a recent paper given at a meeting of the British Association for the Advancement of Science, Dr David Phillipson reported on the current usage of plant-based drugs. His paper was entitled 'The Search for New Drugs from Plants' and in it he explored the idea that plants should be seriously considered, in the search for new drugs.

Dr Phillipson reminds us that we should consider very carefully the economic need to conserve scarce resources. Many synthetic drugs are produced from oil and coal, yet plants need no more than water and carbon dioxide to produce the same, or similar, compounds. One of the statistics quoted by Dr Phillipson was that almost 40 per cent of prescriptions in the United States are for products which contain active ingredients of natural origin. About 25 per cent of all prescription medicines come from plants and 13 per cent from micro-organisms. This proportion has remained very constant over a number of years. On the non-prescription side of medicine he refers to the fact that in America and Europe there is a growing demand for these plant-based drugs. This is sometimes called 'The Green Sweep' – there is in the United Kingdom an estimated 3,000 herbal medicines on sale, containing some 400 herbs, and in Germany the strength of herbal medicine is even more significant. It is obvious that plant-based medicines still play an important part in medicine today and that they possess a very wide range of pharmacological properties.

It is not known just how many types of plants exist in the world, estimates vary from 25,000 up to 500,000. Only a very small number of these have been thoroughly investigated for their chemical structure and ability to act as medicines. In 1975 alone, over 10,000 scientific papers were published on plants for medicinal use. It is clear that there is much more to be learned and it is equally certain that there are within the plant kingdom many more potential drugs which can help to heal all manner of disease.

Further evidence of the interest in herbal medicine in the 1980s can be found in the reports of a World Health Organization symposium on herbal medicine held in Rome in 1979. Delegates from developing countries such as China, Sri Lanka, Egypt, Central Africa,

Mexico and South America gathered together with Western experts to examine the role of health care throughout the world and, in particular, how it would be possible for a system of health care to be made available to all peoples in every land. It was estimated at this symposium that, about 80 per cent of the world's population use herbal remedies.

ECONOMICS OF MEDICINE

It would seem that many herbal remedies which are being used effectively could be made available to more people, freeing the resources needed to produce and develop synthetic drugs for a more effective use. It is believed that, although modern drugs cannot be replaced effectively by herbal remedies in some killer diseases, there is most certainly a case for encouraging the use of herbal remedies in less serious conditions. Much impressive evidence was presented to this conference and the resolution passed at its conclusion called for greater efforts to be made to encourage programmes to widen the use of traditional remedies and, in particular, to make greater use of plants and the remedies of the folk healer and herbalist. Among the diseases which were mentioned as responding to herbal medicines were angina, worms, bronchial asthma, diabetes and many more.

Of course there are many situations where traditional remedies are powerless to treat disease. The great problem facing the world is that modern, effective medicines only work when people can afford to buy and use them and, since many of the poorer nations of the world are not in this position, the World Health Organization are hoping that, by encouraging the use of plant-based medicines, they will be able to save the financial resources devoted to drug research, for investigating only the most serious problems.

DRUG SIDE-EFFECTS

Many people feel great anxiety about the adverse side-effects which result from taking many of these drugs. This is illustrated by a survey reported in the *British Medical Journal* in 1979. This study, carried out over two years, revealed that two out of every five drug prescriptions result in side-effects, many of the side-effects becoming apparent within a matter of days of the treatment commencing. The figures are quite alarming, adverse reactions were experienced by over half the patients taking drugs which affected the central nervous system, such as pain killers and anti-inflammatory agents. Almost as many adverse reactions were experienced by those taking antihistamine drugs which are frequently given to relieve allergies and hay fever. Other drugs with several side-effects, were those used to treat the heart and lungs and antibiotics and drugs taken for stomach and other intestinal problems. The side-effects were so severe in many cases, that those who took the drugs had to discontinue their treatment within three days. The most common side-effects were nausea, diarrhoea, vomiting, headaches, dizziness and general digestive upsets and, in a smaller number of cases, the side-effects were much more serious.

A POPULAR CHOICE

It is not surprising then, that for many people the herbal remedy is the first choice in the treatment of many complaints. Sensibly used, it is a safe and practical method of self-medication and can avoid many of the problems associated with synthetic drugs. With all the latest developments in scientific analysis and control now available to the herbal practitioner, coupled with the long experience of the safe use of herbal medicines, there has never been a safer or better time to use these time-honoured plants in the control and treatment of disease.

Of all the herbal remedies known to man, garlic is without equal. It is an extremely safe medicine, its lack of toxicity having been proved over thousands of years. It is effective in the treatment of all manner of ailments and is the subject of very serious and potentially rewarding areas of research. Even more of the secrets of garlic will be unlocked during the next few years, but what we shall learn is *how* it generates its healing power. The evidence *that* it cures is already with us and has been since man first learned to treat disease.

GLOSSARY

A Glossary of Some Common Herbal Terms

Acrid Having a hot, burning taste or causing heat on the skin.

Active Principle The chemical part of the crude herb that has a healing or beneficial effect.

Alterative An agent which produces a beneficial change in the body without having a marked specific effect.

Analgesic Pain relieving.

Anodyne An agent that soothes pain.

Anthelmintic An agent that expels intestinal worms.

Antibacterial An agent that destroys or suppresses bacteria.

Antibiotic A substance which destroys or stops the growth of micro-organisms.

Anticoagulant A substance that prevents blood or other liquids from clotting.

Antipyretic An agent which helps to reduce high temperature in fever.

Antiseptic A substance which inhibits the growth of micro-organisms.

Antispasmodic A substance which relieves cramps or spasms.

Antitussive A cough-relieving agent.

Aphrodisiac A substance which arouses the sexual instinct.

Astringent An agent which shrinks tissue and restricts discharges.

Carminative A substance which helps to expel gas from the intestines.

Cathartic A strong laxative.

Cholagogue A substance which helps to increase the flow of bile into the intestines.

Colic Acute pain in the abdomen.

Demulcent A substance which soothes irritated tissue particularly mucous membrane.

Diaphoretic A substance which produces perspiration.

Digestive An agent which aids the digestion.

Diuretic A substance which assists the body in disposing of water by promoting urine.

Emetic A substance that causes vomiting.

Expectorant A substance which promotes the discharge of mucus from the respiratory tract.

Febrifuge A fever reducing agent.

Herb A plant having a medicinal, savoury or aromatic property.

Mucilaginous Of a gummy or gelatinous consistency.

Nervine A substance which has a soothing, calming effect on the nerves.

Purgative An agent that produces a powerful laxative effect.

Rubefacient A substance which when applied to the skin causes local irritation and reddening.

Sedative A substance which reduces nervousness, tension and irritation.

Specific Something which cures or relieves a particular condition.

Stomachic A substance which stimulates the stomach, strengthening and toning it.

Tonic A substance which stimulates and strengthens organs or the whole body.

Toxic Poisonous.

Vasodilator An agent which widens the blood vessels.

Vermifuge An agent that expels parasitic worms from the body.

INDEX